The
SUJA JUICE SOLUTION

The
SUJA JUICE
SOLUTION

7 DAYS to Lose Fat, Beat Cravings,
and **Boost Your Energy**

ANNIE LAWLESS
and *JEFF* CHURCH

CO-FOUNDERS *of* SUJA JUICE

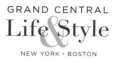

GRAND CENTRAL
Life & Style
NEW YORK · BOSTON

Grand Central Life & Style
Hachette Book Group
1290 Avenue of the Americas
New York, NY 10104

www.GrandCentralLifeandStyle.com

Printed in the United States of America

RRD-C

First Edition: April 2015

10 9 8 7 6 5 4 3 2 1

Grand Central Life & Style is an imprint of Grand Central Publishing.

The Grand Central Life & Style name and logo are trademarks of Hachette Book Group, Inc.

The Hachette Speakers Bureau provides a wide range of authors for speaking events. To find out more, go to www.HachetteSpeakersBureau.com or call (866) 376-6591.

The publisher is not responsible for websites (or their content) that are not owned by the publisher.

Library of Congress Cataloging-in-Publication Data has been applied for.

ISBN: 978-1-455-58927-2

We dedicate this book to all the people
who share our passion for health, wellness,
and living life to its fullest potential, and to our
extended family that now includes—you!

CONTENTS

PART THREE: RECIPES

Juice can change your life. I know this is true, because it absolutely saved mine.

Hi, my name is Annie Lawless. I'm 27 years old and I'm one of the happiest, most energetic, and healthiest people I know!! Yep, double exclamation marks. I'm a certified holistic health and wellness coach, nutritional counselor, avid yogini, and the co-founder of Suja Juice, currently the fastest-growing cold-pressed-beverage company in the United States. My life is on the super-fast track forward and if my enthusiasm sounds excessive or even a tad bit inflated, forgive me, but I'm just so psyched (or *totally juiced*, as we say in the biz) to feel and look as good as I do today—because not so long ago, I didn't look or feel so hot.

Let me explain. As a young girl, I suffered from really awful eczema, allergies, chronic ear infections, and asthma. If you're not familiar with eczema, it's a pretty unsightly rash where the skin becomes inflamed and irritated. And just my not-so-good luck, my eczema wasn't something that flared up occasionally. It appeared daily and faithfully throughout my childhood. I remember way too many slumber parties where I'd have to sneak away to apply gloppy steroid creams

INTRODUCTION

JUICE IS a LIFE CHANGER

to my itchy skin. My skin condition was such a part of my everyday life, I carried tubes of anti-itch cream on me at all times, so that I was armed in the event of attack. I made a habit of wearing long-sleeved shirts and tights or leggings under my school uniform to hide the deep scratches on my arms and legs. Yeah, it was gross and embarrassing, and that was just the eczema.

I was also allergic to *everything*, especially outdoors, where I couldn't last five minutes without having some sort of major reaction. I was constantly sneezing, coughing, or sniffling, and after the steroid cream, Kleenex was my next best friend. Seriously, I was a mess.

Throughout my youth, Mom took me to the pediatrician's office over and over again, but the only solution seemed to be *more* steroid creams, inhalers, or antihistamines. While medicine often helped initially, my faucet nose and scratchy skin always returned with a vengeance. By my preteen years, I was so used to feeling and looking beat-up, I accepted that this was my "normal." It's how I'd always look and feel, and I'd probably be on medications for the rest of my life.

And then one day I went to a new doctor who suggested that my watery eyes, runny nose, and skin rash may actually be an indicator of an autoimmune disease. After several tests, I finally learned that I suffer from lactose intolerance and celiac disease, an immune response to eating gluten, a protein found in wheat, barley, and rye. Today there's a growing awareness about this condition, but at the time *gluten intolerance* was not a term as commonplace as it is now, so I recall thinking I must be seriously ill. *Am I going to die?* My doctor explained that my body was suffering from a severe inflammatory response to dairy and gluten. These substances were acting as foreign invaders in my digestive system that my body couldn't easily defend itself against. In an effort to protect itself, she explained, my body was attacking itself. I had to agree—I had the war wounds to prove it.

To begin the healing process, I was instructed to remove all gluten and dairy from my diet for one week. This meant giving up many of my favorite foods—boxed cereal, peanut butter sandwiches, pasta, and bagels. What was I going to eat? I thought, *Yep, I'm going to die*, but the opposite happened—for the first time I felt like I was actually living. Within seven days of removing gluten and dairy from my diet, the eczema, allergies, and asthma I'd suffered from for my entire life disappeared without a trace. No kidding—I'd never known a life without these nasty conditions, and suddenly they were gone.

I was liberated. After so many years of suffering, I felt like I'd been handed the keys to unlock my highest health potential. I finally understood the direct and powerful correlation between what I put into my body and how I look and feel. For the majority of my life I'd been unknowingly eating foods that were highly irritating to my body, and now I had the knowledge, power, and control to remove them, one by one, and feel and look crazy-good.

My fascination with nutrition was ignited and from that day forward, I embarked on a personal health quest that changed the course of my life. Eventually, I would become a certified health coach, holistic health practitioner, and the co-founder of Suja Juice, but before all that I simply became an overnight health nerd, poring over books on digestion, metabolism, and the properties of natural foods. Truly, I was the only teenager reading *Your Friendly Gut Guide* over summer vacation. Like I said—an A-class nerd. But I didn't care because the more I learned about the basic principles of

nutrition and put them into practice in my own life, the better I felt. Based on my research, I began to develop a new diet and lifestyle for myself where I consciously chose to remove, or "crowd out," not-so-healthy foods and eat only those foods that would rejuvenate my body, rather than slow it down. And that's when juice came into play.

Because I'd spent my entire childhood unintentionally eating foods that aggravated my system, my digestive tract was in major disrepair. The microvilli in my intestinal lining—the finger-like projections on the surface of the intestinal cells that increase the surface area available for absorbing nutrients—were damaged. My body could no longer properly ingest the vital nutrients I needed for optimal health. Even though I'd severely altered my diet by removing gluten and dairy and was consuming fresh fruits, vegetables, healthy fats, and lean meats in abundance, I was still severely vitamin- and nutrient-deficient.

Eager to change my body and open to whatever method would get me there, I began drinking fresh, organic, nutrient-dense juice to replenish my body with the concentrated nutrition I was lacking. What I soon came to understand was how highly efficient juice could be for flooding the body with vital nutrients, minerals, enzymes, phytochemicals, and antioxidants that are easily absorbed into your system.

Because juice contains very little fiber, drinking it requires very little digestive labor. This is a good thing! *Did you know that digestion is the hardest job your body does?* Juice gives your digestive tract a break from the significant energy expenditure required to separate juice from the fiber of whole fruits and vegetables. When you drink pure juice, your body quickly and easily absorbs all of the nutrition from the food because there's no fiber in the way. Fiber, as masterful as it is at regulating and cleaning your digestive tract, can interfere with your body's ability to absorb valuable nutrition.

A medium carrot, for example, has 203 percent of your daily requirement of vitamin A. That's a mega dose! However, that carrot may also contain up to 3 or 4 grams of fiber that cannot be digested by your body. So when you eat that carrot, your body will eliminate much of the indigestible fiber before it has had a chance to absorb and utilize the valuable vitamin A locked inside.

By drinking your fruits and vegetables, you can easily pack 2 or 3 pounds of nutrient-dense natural produce into one 12-ounce glass of juice. That's a lot of digestive enzymes, detoxifying chlorophyll, and concentrated green nutrition that the body can absorb and benefit from without stressing the digestive tract.

I'm the first to admit that I'm kind of an extreme case, but the reality is that most of us—yourself included—could use a bit of help when it comes to getting our digestion back on track, revving up our metabolism, and boosting our nutrition. Over the course of your lifetime, you've likely indulged from time to time in heavily processed, high-in-added-sugars, and not-so-healthy foods. You're human, after all, and a package of Oreos or a basket of chips can be hard for even the most disciplined to resist. You may have also tried to counteract, or reverse, the occasional indulgence by following any number of restrictive diets and weight-loss plans. And unless you live on a remote island or in the far reaches of the planet, you've almost certainly been exposed to environmental pollutants.

All of these factors, individually and collectively, can negatively affect your digestive tract, slow down your metabolism, and create nutrient deficiencies that may alter your overall health and wellness. Even if you're someone who's always eaten healthy, and never experienced any tummy issues that you're aware of, your digestive system has likely still been put through a lot. Again, this is because digestion uses *the most energy* of all the bodily processes. When you think about how many times per day you eat, and how many months and years you've been feeding yourself, you can begin to understand how much digestive labor that is. Your body has been working overtime.

In order to look and feel your best, at some point or another you need to give your digestive system a much-needed break. Giving your digestive system a rest from heavy foods, irritants, and chemicals and replacing them with simple, whole foods and nutrient-, mineral-, and antioxidant-dense juice that can be absorbed into your system with little digestive labor is extremely beneficial—no matter who you are. And once you've given your digestion a chance to flush out the junk, rest, and repair, it can work harder for you than ever.

BABY, IT'S TIME TO SHINE!

If in 7 days of modifying my diet, I felt like a brand-new version of myself, just think how you'll feel after losing a few bad habits and adding high-powered juice and healthier foods to yours. Freakin' A-mazing is the answer. Think about it—by this time next week, you, too, can be the *you* that you've always wanted to be when you start a new job or run into your ex on the street. It's *you* when you're killing it! I mean, who doesn't want that, right?

The health benefits of following the Suja Juice Solution may include:

- Renewed clarity, focus, and energy
- Healthier skin, hair, and nails
- Faster metabolism
- Easier digestion and elimination
- Increased hydration and greater flexibility
- Better sleep
- Reduced hunger and fewer sugar cravings
- Feeling more satisfied and full after meals
- Less fat on your body than a week ago!

The health benefits of the Suja Juice Solution can be extensive and the program is based on the simple diet and lifestyle approach I began to create for myself so many years ago to help heal my digestive sensitivities to gluten and dairy. It's evolved, since then, into an accessible program that can benefit *anyone, whoever you are*. The program you're about to begin hasn't only worked wonders for me. In fact, the Suja Juice Solution has been inspired by juice devotees of all ages, shapes, sizes, and walks of life, including many in the Suja family who have their own transformative 7-day stories (you'll hear from many of them in the pages ahead), and who are equally as passionate and as committed to helping people improve their health and nutrition, one juice at a time.

Take Jeff Church, CEO and co-founder of Suja Juice. His life did a complete 180 once he integrated juice into his life…

Hi, I'm Jeff and I grew up in the Midwest where meals traditionally consist of meat, potatoes, and more meat. When I was first approached by a business colleague and good friend, James Brennan, to grow distribution of a line of green juices that he believed had changed his and his wife's lives, I said, "I don't know. I know juice is hot right now, but drinking it sounds like health with the punishment." I was familiar with the juice craze. I knew it was popular, but really, how much change could adding it to your diet bring about? What could really happen in 7 days? James wouldn't back down, though. At the time, we worked out of the same office space and he'd regularly show up with bottles of earthy green, red, and orange juices he was drinking, and I thought, *No way am I drinking that stuff*. But in an effort to get him off my back, I finally tried one. Wow, it really did stop me in my tracks. I've always stood firm that I'm not willing to eat something just because it's good for me. I'll try anything once, but it has to taste good, too, and this bottle of juice blew me away. I actually liked it. I thought, *Well, if I can enjoy this, anyone can*. What's more, after only a few days of ditching my coffee habit and replacing it with juice, I began to feel…*younger*. More energetic, more focused at work, and like my metabolism had been given a kick in the pants. I took some home for my wife and she soon claimed that after drinking a juice or two throughout the day, she felt more fluid, light, and comfortable in her body. My kids started drinking it, too, and soon they were demanding it instead of soda. This juice—it was the craziest thing.

It wasn't long before I assumed the role of CEO of Suja, and I continue to be amazed by the transformative and restorative power of simple vitamin- and nutrient-dense ingredients. Old habits die hard, so I'm the first to admit that I slip up from time to time (Annie can attest to this!), and when I do eat or drink something less than healthy, I don't beat myself up too much about it because I know how to quickly and easily get back on track. It typically only takes one green juice and a simple, balanced meal before I'm feeling and looking a whole lot better. I continue to be amazed at how these relatively simple changes to my diet have transformed me into the healthiest version of myself. Today Suja is populated by nearly 200 people like Annie and me who share a similar passion for health and wellness, and we're all committed to working every day with a mission of helping even more people like you understand how to significantly shift how you look and feel—*one juice at a time*.

MORE THAN JUICE!

While juice is central to this 7-day program, the refreshing news is that the Suja Juice Solution extends far beyond juice. It's not a severe cleanse or restrictive juice diet where you only drink liquids. This program offers you more. And by more, we mean food! Don't get us wrong—juice cleanses and "detoxes" have their place, and at Suja we've developed several. Many of our celebrity customers love them for how they help them to look and feel before a big premiere or strutting down the red carpet, but a juice cleanse has a hard expiration date. Meaning, it's not a sustainable lifestyle because subsisting on liquids alone isn't how real people live—let alone survive and thrive. Red-carpet moments are just that—*moments*. Sooner than later, the human body not only wants to, but also needs to eat real food.

Did you know that if you're not careful, juice only diets can rob your body of protein, leaving you deficient in the nutrients and materials your body needs? Even more concerning is that if you're not consuming enough calories throughout your all-juice diet, your body will likely start eating lean muscle instead of burning fat for energy. And you know what fat without the muscle looks like—flab!

As with other crash diets that severely limit your fat and caloric intake, the weight you quickly lose on the most restrictive juice cleanses will almost always return to your hips, tummy, and legs as soon as you begin to eat again. This is because you forced your body into starvation mode where your metabolism slows down to a crawl in an effort to conserve calories simply to keep moving. Once you start to eat real foods again, your body goes into a crazy sort of stockpiling mode, storing those extra calories in fat cells it can live on in anticipation of your next hunger strike. Kinda makes you rethink the reward of crash dieting, doesn't it? We take a different approach. The Suja Juice Solution is based on the very approaches used by many of us to maintain and sustain general nutrition and health every day of our lives. As you might expect, it involves a lot of kale and other mighty greens, but it's not all about the juice because we're big believers in sustainable wellness—in other words, setting the foundation, day by sunny day, for a long, beautiful, and healthy life.

To help you get there, the Suja Juice Solution sets you in motion toward establishing healthier dietary habits you can easily sustain for the next 7 days, and for many weeks down the road. It starts with two simple steps—drink nutrient-dense juice in combination with eating healthier whole foods. Yep, it's that simple. Not only that, but as you begin to consume more high-powered vegetable and fruit juice and nutrient-dense fresh foods on a day-to-day basis, you will automatically, and perhaps even unconsciously, crave less of the not-so-great stuff because you're so full of what your body really wants and needs to function at its highest health potential. It may sound too good to be true, but trust us, it happens.

BELIEVE IN YOURSELF

We'll never forget the man who bought 30 bottles of juice on the spot when we did our initial product rollout at Whole Foods Market in La Jolla. William, then in his mid-50s and very overweight, approached us and explained that he was desperately looking for a plan to overhaul his current diet and transform his general health. We suggested he begin drinking low-sugar juices while consciously crowding out a few of his favorite not-so-healthy indulgences (his were potato chips and French fries. What are yours? We all have 'em!) and create meals using simple, whole foods.

Fast-forward to a year later and William resurfaced at another of our product events—but we didn't know it was him at first. An energetic, fit man approached our table and said, "Do you remember me? I bought 30 bottles of your juice when you first came on the market. I became obsessed with juicing soon after that. I started making my own juice blends every day and better managing what and how I eat. I'm within just a few pounds of my goal weight." We were all floored! He looked like a completely different person.

Then there was Claire, a young woman living in Seattle who was seeking a nutrition-based solution to improve the look of her skin. We suggested hydrating and alkalizing green juice and limiting her consumption of refined sugars. Two months later she wrote us back with an attached photo of her beautifully clear and glowing skin. She claimed that once she cut processed sugar from her diet and began drinking natural juice to satisfy her sweet cravings, her skin started to clear up almost overnight. She wrote, "I finally like the face I see back in the mirror."

Finally, we love the sentiments expressed by a good friend of the Suja family, Max Goldberg, the founder of PressedJuiceDirectory .com and LivingMaxwell.com: "I have come to greatly appreciate and understand that what I put into my body needs to support me on both a physical and emotional level. As such, there is nothing that makes me feel so vibrant, happy, and energetic as starting my morning by drinking organic juice. Juicing gives my body the essential nutrients and vitamins that it needs to perform at its best and is critical for helping me maintain a positive and happy outlook. In the past, I used to drink alcohol and do drugs—all to avoid life. I have since given those things up and replaced them with organic juice, which helps me embrace life."

The nutrients, minerals, enzymes, phytochemicals, and antioxidants found in fresh fruit and vegetable juice and whole foods are what our bodies really need to function at their best. And when you give your body what it truly desires, it no longer craves or holds on to what it doesn't. Fed the right ingredients, your body will quickly and quite easily reset itself, *even in just 7 days*.

Part 1

JUICE IS OUR JUICY SECRET

Before you start the week that will radically shift many of your current habits and improve your health and wellness in immeasurable ways, we think it's worth your time to learn a bit more about many of the key health benefits of juicing and why the Suja Juice Solution can work so well. We don't want to bog you down with too much science and overcomplicate the concept of juicing (after all, you're probably anxious to get started), but by understanding how your body reacts to what you put in it, you'll likely be more inspired to fully embrace the program. This knowledge will also help explain the exciting changes to your body every step of the way.

WHAT EXACTLY IS JUICING?

Let's start with the basics. Juicing is extracting the liquid from a fruit or vegetable using either a centrifuge or a press. A centrifugal juicer involves a fast whirring blade that shreds the produce and pushes it through a strainer, yielding the liquid and leaving the pulp in the strainer. A press involves grinding

CHAPTER 1

The SCIENCE BEHIND the SUJA JUICE SOLUTION

No Juicer Required

For our best advice on selecting a juicer, see chapter 5, *Your New Kitchen Tools*. Also, we've included blender-friendly recipes for all the juices in the program for those of you who don't have, or plan on purchasing, a juicer. You can find all juice-to-blended conversions in part 3, *Recipes*.

the produce into a bag, pressing the bag between two plates, and extracting nearly every last drop of the juice out of the pulp.

Both methods of juicing are effective, but in our opinion cold-pressing is nutritionally superior to the centrifugal method, for several reasons. First off, the fast whirring blade in the centrifugal method draws in heat and oxygen, which can damage nutrients, kill valuable enzymes, and cause the juice to oxidize quickly. If you use a centrifugal juicer, aim to consume your juices immediately after juicing to avoid too much nutrient loss from oxidation. If you use a cold press, your juice will keep for longer. Cold-pressed juice can chill in your fridge for up to two days and will retain its deep vibrant color, rich flavor, and vital nutrient density

because it oxidizes at a much slower rate. The cold-pressing method also yields more juice than the centrifugal method because the pulp left in a centrifugal blade is usually still wet (meaning there's still juice in the pulp), while the pulp left over from a cold-press juicer is usually dry—you get nearly every last drop of goodness from the produce used. Because more juice is extracted, fewer fruits and veggies need to be used.

JUICE IS NUTRIENT-DENSE

Juicing fruits and vegetables is a highly effective way to flood the body with vital nutrients in their purest form, including vitamins, minerals, amino acids, electrolytes, and digestive enzymes your body needs to function optimally. This is because juice contains very little fiber. The process of juicing separates the juice from the fiber of the plant, leaving behind the pulp that can often inhibit the absorption of valuable nutrients by the body. When you drink pure juice, your body can quickly and easily absorb much of the nutrition from the food you're consuming and assimilate the vitamins, minerals, enzymes, phytochemicals, and rich chlorophyll throughout your body. It's also an easy way to get more fruits and vegetables into your diet: a 16-ounce juice, without the added water, can pack up to 3 pounds of plant nutrition that you likely wouldn't sit down and eat at once.

Digestion, Absorption, and Elimination

Digestion is the breakdown of food both mechanically (chewing, grinding, mixing) and chemically (digestive enzymes, bile, acids). Absorption comes next and it occurs in the small intestine, which is lined with microvilli—small, finger-like projections that are responsible for absorbing the nutrients from your food. A food that is very easily digested is one very easily absorbed. Fresh fruit and veggie juices fit this bill: They are easily digested and absorbed by the body almost instantly. Once a food has been absorbed in the small intestine, it's assimilated—useful nutrients and chemicals are delivered into the body's cells. Elimination is the final stop where non-useful metabolic waste is excreted via the kidneys, urinary tract, and colon.

- **Enzymes.** When you consume enzyme-dense living plants, digestion begins as soon as your food enters your mouth. By the time your food reaches your stomach, less digestive labor is necessary, giving your body a break from the significant energy expenditure required to break down food. Enzymes in food are destroyed by heat, so by consuming cool or room-temperature enzyme-rich fresh fruit and veggie juices, your body enjoys their maximum benefits.

- **Phytochemicals** are naturally occurring compounds in plants and some of the body's biggest superheroes. There are thousands of phytochemicals—including antioxidants, flavonoids, and carotenoids, like beta-carotene—in different foods we eat. Fruit and veggie juices are extremely rich in these compounds due to their pure concentrated plant content.

- **Electrolytes** are substances containing free ions that conduct electricity. All life-forms, including humans, need electrolytes to survive. Sodium, potassium, and magnesium are three common electrolytes that muscles, including the heart, need in order to contract. When electrolytes are imbalanced, your body is imbalanced. Water does not contain electrolytes, but fruit and veggie juices are very rich in electrolytes and can help maintain a healthy balance of sodium, potassium, and magnesium in the body while also providing hydration, vitamins, and minerals.

- **Amino acids** are the raw materials that work with enzymes to build muscles, blood, and organs, and to produce hormones. They play a role in many body functions and systems including digestion and assimilation of foods, cell renewal, and liver function. Deficiencies can cause poor digestion. All juices contain easily digested amino acids, and greens and sprouts have the highest content.

- **Chlorophyll** is the green pigment in plants and is a very alkaline, or neutralizing, substance. Because our bodies tend to be acidic from the overconsumption of processed foods, dairy, coffee, soda, and sugar, alkalizing juice can help neutralize that acidity and bring our pH levels back

into balance. Chlorophyll-dense foods can also help to relieve constipation by breaking up toxic matter in the colon.

JUICE IS A GREAT NEUTRALIZER

Your pH balance is the measurement between acid and alkaline in the body. Ideally, your pH should land somewhere around 7.4, which is slightly alkaline. While it's most beneficial to consume both acid and alkaline foods to maintain a healthy equilibrium in the body, the American diet is generally more acidic than alkaline, which means many of us are experiencing a pH imbalance that can lead to any number of health problems. For example, a pH imbalance in the body has been linked to digestive issues like heartburn, bloating, and constipation. Not a very healthy feeling!

To correct your pH imbalance and move your body back toward a healthy equilibrium, it's important to shift your diet toward more alkaline than acidic foods, which is exactly what the Suja Juice Solution does. Every day, you will consume juices that contain a concentrated dose of highly alkaline greens. You will also be eating whole-food meals high in neutralizing fruits and veggies, healthy fats and oils, and gluten-free grains. At the same time, you will crowd out some of the most acidic foods like dairy, sugar, soy, processed foods, caffeine, and alcohol. Note: The aim of this program is not to alkalize your consumption entirely, but to create meals where 75 to 80 percent of your plate is alkaline and the other 20 to 25 percent is acidic.

JUICE HELPS TO FLUSH OUT WASTE

The Suja Juice Solution is designed to reset your body to a cleaner, more balanced state by flushing out waste—processed food residues, irritants, and pollutants that have built up, often as physical weight, over time. By crowding out your consumption of less-than-healthy, difficult-to-digest foods and crowding in pure, nutrient-dense juice and alkalizing whole foods, you allow your body to begin the important process of reducing waste because, quite simply, you've stopped piling more junk on top of the heap. Additionally,

when the body is clean and has the nutrition it needs to function as intended, the removal of waste and weight happens easily and naturally because the digestive organs are supported in doing their jobs efficiently.

Many of the foods that you will be crowding out over the course of this program are considered wasteful—that is, "filled with waste"—because they introduce into the body foreign chemicals, particles, and pollutants that cannot be digested and eliminated properly, so they are stored in the tissues and blood and interfere with natural processes. In particular, the elimination organs and the body's digestion and metabolism cannot function optimally if the body is clogged up with this stuff. Waste that sits in the intestines for too long can lead to bloating, constipation, weight gain, and even malabsorption, where the intestine has difficulty absorbing nutrients from food. Improperly eliminated waste can also compromise healthy intestinal bacteria causing brain fog, sluggishness, and fatigue.

The alkaline, mineral-dense qualities of fresh, hydrating juices nourish and support the function of the digestive organs— the pancreas, small and large intestines, gallbladder, and liver, which are all vital for performing crucial metabolic functions in the body, including the digestion of fat. Certain juices—carrot, for example, with its high levels of beta-carotene and numerous other carotenes like lutein and lycopene—are especially supportive to the liver. Beta-carotene is converted to vitamin A in the body, where it is believed to act as a potent antioxidant that attacks free radicals. Vitamin A is also believed to reduce fat in the liver, which helps to detoxify the body.

JUICE BENEFITS YOUR IMMUNE SYSTEM

Certain vitamins and minerals are crucial to a healthy immune system. These include zinc, selenium, iron, vitamins A, C, and E, folic acid, vitamin B_6, and copper. A deficiency in these nutrients, even a slight one, can impair a healthy immune response. Not only is the typical American diet lacking in many of these key vitamins, minerals, and nutrients, but many of the processed foods we eat (which are high in sugar, salt, unnatural fats, and chemicals) further compromise the immune system. Juicing fresh, whole, organic fruits and vegetables is an effective immune-supporting practice because they're nutrient-dense; they provide the body's immune system with much of the nutrition it needs to respond appropriately. Over the course of this program, you will maximize the juice that floods the body with concentrated nutrition while minimizing foods and substances that compromise your immune system.

A Nourishing Drink

Juice itself is not a magic bullet. It does not melt away pounds or reverse the aging process. What juice *does* do is nourish the body so your organs can function properly, efficiently, and at peak performance. Fresh fruit and vegetable juices contain extremely valuable concentrated vitamins, minerals, and enzymes that support healthy immune system function, digestion, and metabolic functions.

JUICE CURBS CRAVINGS

The Suja Juice Solution is designed to fill you up with concentrated plant nutrition and hydration, reducing many of your cravings for processed, oily, sugary, and salty foods. Did you know that dehydration is often mistaken for hunger, and that in many instances, a hunger craving is the result of a vitamin, mineral, or nutrient deficiency? For example, if you aren't getting enough magnesium, you might be craving chocolate. If you aren't getting enough iron, you might be craving a burger. If you aren't getting enough omega-3 fatty acids, you might be craving salty potato chips. If you aren't getting enough calcium, you might be craving ice cream. When you nourish your body with what it truly needs, it's not left craving or wanting more, because it's been properly fed. The Suja Juice Solution uses juice to both hydrate and nourish your body with essential nutrients. Used in this way, it becomes a powerful catalyst toward making better food choices and diminishing cravings—most notably the craving for sugar.

Sugar is America's biggest contributor to obesity and diabetes, and recent studies have suggested that the chemical reactions that sugar creates in the brain are more addictive than drugs like heroin and cocaine. The majority of us can probably attest that the more we eat the sweet stuff, the more we want it. Unfortunately, because sugar is in so many of the foods we consume—often without our even realizing it—this creates a cycle of addiction and overconsumption of unnatural

"Sugar" Goes By Many Names

Agave	High-fructose corn syrup
Artificial sweeteners	Honey
Barley malt	Lactose
Beet sugar	Malt syrup
Brown rice syrup	Maltodextrin
Brown sugar	Maple syrup
Cane sugar	Molasses
Carob syrup	Oat syrup
Coconut sugar	"Raw" sugar
Corn syrup	Refined white sugar
Date sugar	Sorghum
Evaporated cane juice	Sucanat
Fruit juice concentrate	Tapioca syrup
Glucose	Turbinado sugar

quantities and forms. (Just start reading food labels and you'll soon recognize that sugar, in some form or another, is ubiquitous.)

So how do we begin to curb our cravings for sugar, and the nearly inevitable addiction to it?

You can start now by eating less processed sugar and incorporating pure juice into your diet.

When you crowd out processed, concentrated, and refined sugars with the natural sugars contained in pure juice (unprocessed fructose and glucose), you satisfy your craving for sweetness. At the same time, your body can easily absorb and efficiently metabolize the natural, unprocessed sugars in juice and use them for energy right away.

JUICE + WHOLE FOOD = SUSTAINABLE HEALTH

To function at its highest health potential, your body needs a balanced combination of proteins, fats, and carbohydrates from a variety of food sources. This is why the Suja Juice Solution is not a juice-only program but one that deliberately combines fresh juices with whole foods. While the program is juice-centric (we are juice makers, after all), the juices and tonics you'll be drinking over the course of the next 7 to 28 days will benefit your body most when consumed in combination with the recommended foods. The juices have been carefully designed by Bryan Riblett, a graduate of the Culinary Institute of America and head of innovation for Suja, and the whole-food meals have been created by Annie Lawless, nutritional counselor and co-founder of Suja. The juices + whole-food meals work together to optimally stimulate the digestion, absorption, and assimilation of supercharged nutrition throughout your body, along with the elimination of unusable waste. Included in the pages ahead are 75 of our favorite family recipes for morning, midday, and early-evening juice + whole-food meals, plus ideas for grab 'n' go snacks, desserts, spirits, and everything you need to know to make your own Suja juices at home. We've also included 30-plus bonus-hydration recipes for when you're craving something extra juicy.

With the science out of the way, it's time to begin to experience the epic taste and nutritional benefits of the Suja Juice Solution.

There are just two simple steps to this program:

Step 1. Add three nutrient-dense juices every day.

Step 2. Crowd out not-so-healthy foods with fresh, whole foods.

That's it. The Suja Juice Solution is a simple two-step hydration- and whole-food-centered plan created to give you the nutrition your body truly craves and needs through high-powered, pure juice and an array of wholesome, organic fruits and vegetables, whole grains, healthy fats, and lean proteins.

STEP 1. DRINK YOUR JUICE

As you learned in the last chapter, *The Science Behind the Suja Juice Solution*, juicing fruits and vegetables is a highly effective and efficient way to flood and replenish your body with the minerals, enzymes, vitamins, amino acids, antioxidants, electrolytes, and chlorophyll that are vital to a healthy digestive tract, eliminating waste, and resetting

CHAPTER 2

HOW the SUJA JUICE SOLUTION WORKS

> ### Did You Know—Not All Greens Are Created Equal?
>
> The corner salad bar doesn't look the way it used to. Iceberg lettuce is out, and kale and chard are in! Not only are dark leafy greens more substantive and filling than limp lettuce, but they're also nutritionally superior. Dark leafy greens are rich in some of the nutrients most deficient in the American diet, including magnesium, vitamin D, and iron. As soon as you make the switch to dark leafy greens, you'll begin to reap the nutritional benefits.

your body to a more balanced state. It's also a convenient and fairly easy way to consume the fruits and veggies your body needs every day to maintain overall health. It can feel like a challenge, and sometimes even a chore, to eat enough greens every day—especially if you're traveling, working long hours, driving kids to and from school, or just generally busy and on the go with limited access to fresh produce and time for all-out cooking. Juicing makes it convenient to pack, or sneak, multiple servings of nutrient-dense fruits and vegetables onto your daily plate. (Most of us don't make a practice of devouring two

or three heads of raw kale at every meal, nor could we easily chew and digest it!) Juicing also creates an opportunity to combine what are sometimes bitter, dark leafy greens with sweet, fragrant fruits in a way that is both healthful *and* satisfying.

STEP 2. CROWD OUT

As you begin to feel the power of the concentrated green nutrition you're bringing into your body each day, we encourage you to crowd out not-so-healthy foods (we'll explain how particular "out-crowd" foods slow you down in just a bit) while maximizing healthier, high-quality foods that will get you to looking and feeling your best—faster.

HOW DO I DO THIS?

The Suja Juice Solution starts with a powerful 7-day reset program, which floods your body with essential vitamins, minerals, and nutrients and gives you fast, feel-good results. By enabling your body to efficiently hydrate and flush out waste by providing it with proper nourishment, you can expect to have more energy and mental focus, experience better digestion, and see a decrease in water weight. Yes, you'll likely lose unwanted fat, too, all in just 7 days. After the 7-day reset, you're invited to extend the program to a full 28 days for maximum benefit and results, including an easy-to-follow maintenance plan that can be tailored just for you and your lifestyle.

While the extended 28-day Suja Juice Solution is optional, we do recommend that if this is your first time following the program you renew your commitment beyond the first 7 days. Here's why: Quickly returning to your eating and lifestyle habits after 7 days of rebalancing your body with clean nourishment can shock your system, upsetting that delicate balance you've just reset. Also, while many not-so-healthy habits can most definitely be shifted in one week, healthier habits can be formed when you extend the program for a longer period of time. By continuing with the program for a full 28 days and adding replenishing foods back onto your plate—slowly and one at a time—you move closer to establishing a healthy equilibrium that will be easy (and perhaps even breezy!) for you to sustain for months and years ahead.

A SLOW AND STEADY BUILD

After the initial 7-day reset, the program slowly builds on itself. Week to week, your juice and whole-food options increase and the nutritional benefits to your body expand exponentially so that by the end of the full 28 days, you're likely to feel even more rested, energetic, and focused. You may notice that your skin looks more plump and hydrated. It may even begin to brighten, clear, and almost glow. You might also experience less stiffness in your body and more ease in your movements. And finally, you're likely to have far fewer sugar cravings (if any!), a shift in appetite, and an even slimmer waistline. Celebrate—the benefits are endless!

PROGRAM SNEAK PEAK

We give you all of the day-to-day details you need to follow the Suja Juice Solution beginning in part 2 of the book, including 75 of our favorite family recipes and everything you need to know to make your own juices at home or quickly order on the go, but here's a brief overview of the way the program works—a sneak peak of what's ahead:

- Days 1–7 Reset Program

- Days 8–14 to Reinforce

- Days 15–21 to Recharge

- Days 22–28 to Renew

7 DAYS TO RESET: REBALANCE

For 7 days, you will consume three fresh, organic juices a day that will provide the healthful hydration and nourishment your body needs, while also enabling your body to eliminate waste, and rebalance to a healthier state. In addition, you will consume three gentle and easily digestible "reset" meals a day (recipes included) that work harmoniously with the juices included in the program. As you flood your body with a complete range of plant-based hydration and whole-food nutrition, including key vitamins, minerals, and electrolytes in addition to nourishing proteins, natural fats, and complex

carbohydrates, you're encouraged to crowd out the foods that tend to stall you along the path toward vibrant health. These foods include:

Out-Crowd Foods

(See chapter 3 for more information and a full list of these out-crowd foods.)

Grains (including gluten-free)

Legumes and peanuts

High-starch veggies

Refined and added sugars

Dried fruits

Red meat

Lunch meat

Dairy

Hydrogenated and partially hydrogenated oils

Soy products

Processed foods

Caffeine

Alcohol

Gulp. If parting with your morning coffee and bowl of O's feels like major punishment even for a day, don't despair—you will see them at the breakfast table again. After

7 days, you're invited to welcome many of these foods back into your life. Nothing is off the menu forever. But, for the purposes of resetting your body and giving your digestive system a break, we encourage you to crowd them out for a solid week, and then check in with yourself and notice how you feel. Once you've given yourself a chance to experience a week without them, you may discover that you look and feel a whole lot better, and that life without many of these out-crowd foods isn't punishment at all. Imagine that!

7 DAYS TO REINFORCE: FORTIFY YOUR MOTIVATION FOR A CLEANER LIFESTYLE

Assuming you feel awesome—looking and feeling better than you have in years—we invite you to keep the good feelings going. Why stop now when you can extend the program for optimal health and wellness? During the reinforce week, as you slowly add foods back onto your plate, you will begin to replenish your body and fortify your motivation and commitment to looking and feeling *even better*.

Here's how the reinforce week works: Every day you will drink three juices (morning, midday, and early evening) and eat three whole-food meals in between. You will continue to eat simple clean foods, but this week you can *add back* onto your plate a variety of foods you spent the last 7 days living without—foods like legumes, low-glycemic whole fruits, some starchy veggies, along with healthy fats—to give you that extra get-up-and-go.

For simplicity and ease, the whole-food meal recipes build on each other from one week to the next, becoming more and more flavorful, colorful, and filling. In fact, you may not even realize that the new dishes you're creating utilize many of the same simple ingredients from a week ago, which makes cooking them a breeze. What we've discovered is that the key to good cooking is to start with fresh, healthy ingredients and simply combine them. It's not that complicated!

7 DAYS TO RECHARGE: SHIFT YOUR FOCUS FROM REMOVAL TO REPLENISHMENT

This week, you will shift your focus from elimination and removal to replenishment, consuming juices and whole-food combinations that fuel your body, satisfy your cravings, and recharge you with abundant energy.

This next round of 7 days builds upon the last. Every day you will be encouraged to drink three juices and eat three whole-food meals in between. In addition to preparing heartier and more complex meal recipes, you'll also be invited to add a snack and a satisfying dessert to your day. You'll continue to crowd out the slowest of the slow-down foods—like refined sugars, alcohol, and processed foods—while reintroducing healthy, gluten-free grains, tropical fruits, grass-fed meats, goat's and sheep's dairy—plus caffeine and some natural sugars. This week, as you add more complex foods back onto your plate, you'll have the opportunity to reflect on which foods satisfy and recharge you the most, and which foods you're content to continue to go without.

7 DAYS TO RENEW: RENEW YOUR COMMITMENT TO A LONG BEAUTIFUL LIFE

In the final 7 days of the program, you're invited to eat as you normally do—and by this time you may discover that you have a *new normal*. In addition to your regular meals, you'll add three delicious, organic juices—one before each of your three meals. It's not required that you crowd out any foods, just make your preferred choices, meal by meal, and our bet is that you'll notice that by your own choosing you'll make healthier, more natural food choices that help you feel and look your best. This is precisely the goal of the program and our shared dream for you. By the end of the 28 days you will have created a nutritional and lifestyle plan that you can, and very much want to, sustain into the days, weeks, months, and years ahead.

Whether you follow the Suja Juice Solution for a full 28 days or prefer the shorter 7-day reset, you will experience the most feel-better results when in addition to flooding your body with concentrated juice nutrition, you crowd out less-than-healthy foods and crowd in healthier, high-quality foods. This simple action will get you to looking and feeling your best—faster. Turn the page now for a detailed breakdown of what foods provide your body with the vitamins and minerals it needs daily to function optimally and help you reach your highest health potential.

The Suja Juice Solution is a hydration- and whole-food-centered plan created to eliminate anything that can wreak havoc on your digestive system, slow down your metabolism, create unhealthy cravings, and basically contribute to less-than-optimal health. For these reasons we strongly suggest crowding out the following foods for the first 7 days of the reset program to make more room for the high-powered juice and clean nutrition that will be flooding and filling up your body with 100 percent goodness.

EAT LESS OF THESE OUT-CROWD FOODS

Grains (Including Gluten-Free Grains)

How grains can slow you down:
Bloating, fat storage, brain fog, fatigue

Grains can be difficult for the body to break down and digest, especially hybridized wheat. With grains crowded out from your diet for the first 7 days of the Suja Juice Solution, you may notice that you experience less hunger and more energy. Why? Grains elicit a greater insulin response than other foods because they're concentrated carbohydrates that when digested are reduced to glucose, or simple sugar. A rush of sugar in the bloodstream can cause a blood sugar spike and subsequent fall. You know, that uncomfortable crash-and-burn feeling? When your blood sugar crashes from a roller-coaster high, your body tends to crave more sugar in an effort to lift it back up. Feeding this machine can easily lead to overeating, weight gain, and fatigue.

Combining grains with a healthy fat or lean protein will slow down the body's digestion time and minimize a radical blood sugar response, but consider that about 50 grams of carb (a modest bowl of quinoa or brown rice) is still going to be reduced to simple sugar, and if the sugar from those grains isn't immediately used as energy or to replenish glycogen stores, the body stores it as fat. So for the first 7 days of the reset program, skip the grains and fill up on healthier in-crowd foods—which can often leave you feeling *more* satisfied than bread, crackers, or pasta.

> ➤ *CROWD OUT THESE GRAINS:*
> **All, including gluten-free: wheat, rye, barley, spelt, kamut; and gluten-free amaranth, brown rice, buckwheat, hemp seed, millet, quinoa, and whole or steel-cut oats**

White Flour

How white flour can slow you down:
Blood sugar spikes, hunger, weight gain

White flour is a highly processed and refined form of wheat. It has been stripped of all its nutrients and fiber, which is why most white flour is "fortified." Synthetic vitamins and minerals are added back in to give it some nutritional value, but white flour really does nothing for your body except reduce very quickly to glucose, a simple sugar that can spike your blood sugar much the way grains do. This triggers a rapid insulin release and a hormone response to store the excess sugar as fat.

> ➤ *CROWD OUT THESE WHITE FLOUR FOODS:*
> **Bagels and rolls, pastries and baked goods, cereal, crackers, white bread**

Legumes

How legumes can slow you down:
Bloating, poor digestion

Beans contain lectins, which are a natural anti-nutrient protein that can cause digestive stress. Beans are also a complex combination of protein, carbohydrate, and fiber, so they can be difficult for the body to break down and digest. When a food isn't easily digested, your body cannot absorb and assimilate nutrients and eliminate it efficiently. This can create bloating and you know what else! After the 7-day reset, you can add whole beans back into your diet as a great source of vegetarian protein and fiber, but removing them all, with the exception of lentils, from the beginning stages of the program will give your digestion a chance to rest and reset.

> ➤ *CROWD OUT THESE LEGUMES:*
> **Black beans, butter beans, cannellini beans, chickpeas, great northern beans, kidney beans, lima beans, navy beans, pinto beans, refried beans (all), white beans**

Peanuts

How peanuts can slow you down:
Highly allergenic, poor digestion

Did you know that peanuts actually aren't nuts? They're legumes, and as you just learned—legumes are difficult to digest. In addition, most peanuts for mainstream consumption are stored in mass quantities in facilities where mold is prevalent. According to the U.S. National Library of Medicine, while storage methods have improved in the United States, mold is still so common that the FDA has declared it an "unavoidable contaminant" in peanut production. Peanuts are also highly allergenic and can cause tummy pain, gas, nausea, and diarrhea, although you don't have to be allergic to peanuts to suffer from digestive difficulty.

High-Starch Veggies

How high-starch foods can slow you down:
Blood sugar spikes, fat storage

Similar to grains and white flour, high-starch veggies can trigger a blood sugar spike, which is potentially problematic for rebalancing and resetting your system. While they do contain essential vitamins, antioxidants, and valuable fiber and are a great source of energy, they're removed from the first 7 days of the reset program to help reduce your sugar cravings and to give your taste buds a chance to reset. They're one of the first foods you're invited to add back onto your plate, although after a week of replacing them with a delicious array of non-starchy veggies (which are lower in natural sugar and calories), you may discover a new appreciation for the simpler things in life.

> ► *CROWD OUT THESE HIGH-STARCH VEGGIES:*
> Beets, carrots, corn, green garden peas, sugar snap peas, sweet potatoes, white potatoes, winter squash (butternut, acorn, kabocha, pumpkin, hubbard, delicata, spaghetti), yams

Refined and Non-Fruit Sugar

How sugar can slow you down:
Increased cravings, weight gain, disruptions to cognition and the immune system, skin aging

It's a fact—refined and processed sugars are bad news, and they're some of the most overused food additives in our country. Sugars are everywhere—crackers, cereal, salad dressing, yogurt, lunch meat, bread, soup, sauces, and on and on. In addition to being addictive and intensifying your sweet cravings, processed sugars and even some natural sugars like agave can be a metabolic nightmare because they elicit a violent insulin release into the bloodstream to quickly balance the body's elevated blood sugar levels. And if that weren't enough of a reason to stay away from the sweet stuff, sugar can age your skin through a process called glycation that damages collagen and elastin in the skin. This can lead to wrinkling, sagging, and general dullness. So stick to the low-glycemic fruit and veggie juices as your sweet source in the first 7 days of the reset program. Eventually you'll be invited to add back and enjoy mineral-rich natural sweeteners like maple syrup, honey, and coconut sugar—all of which have unique and wonderful flavors on their own as well as a more balanced effect on your blood sugar level. Note: The one sweetener you can use throughout the program is stevia, a naturally derived sweetener that comes from the stevia plant and doesn't spike your blood sugar level.

> ► *CROWD OUT THESE ADDED SUGARS:*
> Artificial sweeteners (all), cane sugars (white sugar, brown sugar, evaporated cane juice, "raw" sugar, turbinado sugar, sucanat, sucrose), corn syrup and high-fructose corn syrup, natural sweeteners (agave, beet sugar, brown rice syrup, coconut sugar, date sugar, honey, maple syrup, molasses)

Did You Know Agave Ain't So Sweet?

Contrary to conventional wisdom, agave nectar is not a healthy sugar substitute. It's made up of more fructose than any other added sweetener (70 to 98 percent). To put this in perspective, highly processed high-fructose corn syrup, HFCS, has significantly less fructose (55 percent) than agave nectar. While fructose is a natural sugar, in agave nectar it's in an unnaturally concentrated form that is very difficult for your body to metabolize efficiently. Fructose, like alcohol, is entirely broken down in the liver and directly converted to the type of fat that is stored in the belly.

Whole Fruit

How whole fruit can slow you down:
Elevated blood sugar levels, overeating, fat storage

Let's be clear—fruits are a wonderful source of hydration and are rich in valuable minerals, vitamins, and enzymes, plus they are nutritious sources of fuel for the body and brain. We love fruits! However, fruit does contain naturally occurring sugars (glucose and fructose), and while natural sugars are our favorite kind, it can be very easy to consume more than you need to fuel your body. With the exception of low-glycemic citrus fruits (lemons, limes, and grapefruit) that help to flush out unusable waste by stimulating natural enzymes, we ask that you cut down on your whole-fruit intake in the first 7 days of the reset program to help dial down your sweet tooth and reset your sensitivity to natural sweetness. By limiting your fruit intake to the fresh juices you're making daily, you will consume an appropriate amount of natural sugars to fuel your activity levels without disrupting your blood sugar levels and slowing down your metabolism.

> ➤ *CROWD OUT THESE WHOLE FRUITS:*
> All, except lemons, limes, grapefruit, tomatoes, and avocado

Dried Fruit

How dried fruit can slow you down:
Elevated blood sugar levels, overeating, fat storage, dehydration

Dried fruits are whole fruits with all their water removed. They contain extremely concentrated amounts of fruit sugar (fructose and glucose); if these aren't quickly burned as energy, they're stored as excess sugars in your fat cells. It's easy to overeat dried fruits because they've been drastically reduced in volume. It's a cinch to pop a handful of dried apricots into your mouth, whereas you'd typically not consume five whole apricots in one sitting. Dried fruits are also difficult for the body to digest because their texture is so tough and dry. They contain no water content to hydrate the small intestine and move things along. The body must rehydrate them in order to digest them, which is extremely dehydrating. Ever notice how dried fruit makes you thirsty?

Red Meat

How red meat can slow you down:
Exposure to pollutants, difficult digestion

Much of the conventionally produced red meat available in grocery stores—any meat that's not certified organic or grass-fed—can contain hormones, chemicals, and antibiotics that can prevent us from developing a healthy immune system. Additionally, red meat often contains pro-inflammatory fatty acids, which can aggravate the body in a number of ways. Red meat also produces an acidic by-product called uric acid that can be hard on your kidneys to process. When your kidneys are feeling stressed, they cannot effectively do what they do best—release and flush out waste. While red meat can be an excellent source of protein and iron, we recommend that you crowd it out of your diet for the first 7 days of the program in an effort to give your body the opportunity it needs to rest and reset to a cleaner state.

➤ *CROWD OUT THESE RED MEATS:*
Bacon (beef, pork, and turkey), beef, bison, duck, game meats, lamb, pork, rabbit, sausage

Lunch Meat

How lunch meat can slow you down:
Water retention, bloating, consumption of nitrates

We believe fresh is best, so packaged lunch meats are not our ideal choice for you. Many contain high-fructose corn syrup that's often stored as fat, and massive amounts of sodium that can cause water retention and bloating and put you well over your recommended daily salt intake. Another common additive in lunch meats is nitrate, which is used to manage the growth of bacteria and extend shelf life by slowing down the breakdown of fat in the meat. As you might guess, ingesting nitrates can also slow *you* down. While many grocers and natural food stores now carry nitrate-free lunch meat, skip the turkey sandwiches for the first 7 days of the reset program as you focus instead on eating foods that help to speed up your metabolism, rather than stall it.

Dairy

How dairy can slow you down:
Allergies, poor digestion, congestion

Due to its high content of animal-based fat and lactose (naturally occurring milk sugar), dairy can bring the body to a near standstill. Skim and fat-free aren't any better. In fact, these low-calorie versions can slow your digestion down even more than full fat. The high percentage of people who suffer from lactose intolerance is a strong indicator that the human body generally lacks the appropriate digestive enzymes for cow's milk. Additionally, many conventionally raised dairy cows are pumped with growth hormones and antibiotics that may be disruptive to our natural hormone levels and overall health. Conventionally raised cows are also often fed low-grade food containing GMOs. Genetically modified organisms are plants or animals that have been genetically engineered with DNA from different species (including bacteria and viruses) to create a mix of genes that do not traditionally occur or resemble anything in nature.

In addition to all this, much of the milk you find on the shelves has been pasteurized—heated to a high temperature and swiftly cooled before packaging. While pasteurization of milk can destroy harmful bacteria and pathogenic microbes in addition to extending shelf life, the process can also compromise valuable enzymes, vitamins, and protein.

> ➤ *CROWD OUT THESE DAIRY FOODS:*
> **Calcium supplements (with whey or lactose), casein, cheese, cream, cream cheese, ice cream, kefir, lactose-containing foods or products, milk, puddings, sour cream, whey-containing products, yogurt**

Bad Fats

How bad fats can slow you down:
Difficult digestion, high cholesterol

Most vegetable oils are highly processed, heated to temperatures as high as 500°F, and made from genetically engineered crops created to withstand pesticides, produce more oil, and grow bigger. The result of all this heavy-duty processing is that the plants are mutated into a denatured state and into a fat the body does not easily recognize or digest. Think about it: When an oil (say, cottonseed oil—which is oil made from cotton) goes through a heavy manufacturing process, a food product is created that doesn't resemble the natural state of the plant. Hydrogenated oils are the most denatured of them all. They are created by adding hydrogen atoms to a double bond in the oil, increasing the saturated fat level by converting the type of bond to a "trans" bond. What does all this mad science mean? Hydrogenated oil, otherwise known as trans-fats, are completely foreign to the body and are considered by many doctors to be the worst type of fat you can ingest. Trans-fats have been linked to high cholesterol and hardening of the artery walls, among other ailments.

> ➤ *CROWD OUT THESE BAD FATS:*
> **Canola oil, corn oil, cottonseed oil, grapeseed oil, hydrogenated or partially hydrogenated oils (all), margarine, peanut oil, rice bran oil, safflower oil, soybean oil, sunflower oil**

Soy Products

How soy can slow you down:
Disrupts estrogen levels in men and women; hard to break down, metabolize, and digest; can create belly fat

Over 90 percent of soy in the United States is genetically modified, according to the USDA, which means the seeds for most soy crops are made in a lab. Soy also contains phytoestrogens, which is bad news for your hormones; consuming large quantities of soy has been linked to estrogen disruption, slow metabolism, and weight gain. Most soy products are highly processed—boiled, strained, hydrolyzed, and isolated into powder, which creates a food product your body doesn't recognize and often doesn't know what to do with. For example, most energy bars, protein powders, and smoothie drinks contain soy protein isolate. This is one of the most refined soy products you can consume. It's created by heating soybeans to a very high temperature, stripping them of everything except their protein, and milling it into an isolated powder. Long story short, you won't find soy protein isolate hanging on a tree, and your body definitely won't recognize it or know how to digest it properly.

> ➤ *CROWD OUT THESE SOY FOODS AND PRODUCTS:*
> **Edamame, soybean oil, soy cheese, soy meats, soy milk, soy protein powders, soy yogurt, tempeh, tofu**

Processed Foods

How processed foods can slow you down:
Poor digestion, weight gain

If it has more than five ingredients that you cannot pronounce and comes in a box, bag, or can, it's probably processed. Processed foods—including packaged cookies and cake, cereal, instant oatmeal, crackers, chips, bread, bagels, dips, salad dressings, frozen foods, and fast foods—are typically full of preservatives, sugars, sodium, and other additives. Many of them taste good, but most of us intuitively know processed foods are not exactly "foods." Real foods found in nature do not need any processing, nor do they contain 25 ingredients. An ear of corn grows on a farm, but high-fructose corn syrup does not. A tomato may be found in nature, but ketchup is not. A stalk of wheat grows from a seed, but cereal does not. You get the picture. The more processed a food is, the less natural it becomes, and the human body is not designed to digest these complicated, often chemical-heavy foods that are relatively new to the food chain. Our bodies haven't developed the digestive system, enzymes, and processes to break them down efficiently. When the body cannot properly digest, assimilate, and eliminate foods, it will store them as waste—in other words, weight!

Caffeine

How caffeine can slow you down:
Dehydration, fatigue, mood swings, hormone disruption

Caffeine is a stimulant, and like most stimulants it sets you up for an inevitable crash. Caffeine swings can dramatically affect your mood and level of energy—all of which can lead to overeating. Caffeine can stress your adrenal gland, which regulates the hormone aldosterone, which in turn controls efficient sugar storage and fat metabolism. Your morning cup of coffee or black tea also increases the release of the stress hormone cortisol. Does coffee ever make you anxious? This is why! Before starting the first 7 days of the reset program, we suggest you taper off caffeine (more on how to kick your caffeine habit in chapter 6), and then in an effort to rebalance your body, we ask that you take a complete break from caffeine on day 1 of the reset program. Take note—this is a break, not a *breakup*. You will eventually be invited to bring caffeine back into your life, if you so choose, and savor it in moderation.

> ➤ *CROWD OUT THESE SOURCES OF CAFFEINE:*
> **Black tea, chocolate, coffee, decaf coffee, pain relievers with caffeine (Excedrin migraine), soda**

Alcohol

How alcohol can slow you down:
Sluggish metabolism, hard on the liver

Alcohol stresses the important metabolizing and detoxifying function of the liver, so it is crowded out for the first 21 days of this program to allow your body to fully eliminate waste and weight without interference. If your liver is working to metabolize alcohol, it cannot focus its energy elsewhere. That's why we suggest you crowd out alcohol for the first few weeks of the program to show your liver some love and let it work as hard as it can for you.

Additionally, many alcohols are grain-based, which you're sending on vacation as well, along with processed and added sugars that are prevalent in many mixed drinks and cocktails. Without you even realizing it, you can consume hundreds of empty sugary calories at one cocktail party. This doesn't mean the fun is over. By week 4, the renew week, you're invited to indulge (responsibly) again.

That's it. End of out-crowd list. Think you can live without these foods for 7 days? We bet you can do almost *anything* for 7 days, so you've easily got this. Plus, consider that when you're beginning each of your meals by drinking delicious, fresh, and satisfying juice, you will naturally start to crowd out many of these foods without thinking much about it or feeling deprived, as you crowd *in* the healthier foods.

EAT MORE OF THESE IN-CROWD FOODS

Time for you to meet the "in" crowd. For the first 7 days of the reset program, fill your plate with the following healthful, nutritious, and delicious whole foods and ingredients.

Leafy Greens

How greens can make you shine: As far as we're concerned, leafy greens are 100 percent goodness. They contain beneficial fiber, enzymes, protein, minerals, and antioxidants. They're also extremely rich in vitamins and chlorophyll, which helps oxygenate the blood. Add to that, dark leafy greens are low in sugar and calories, so you can eat as much as you want and feel good about flooding your body with the best source of plant-based nutrition available. What else can we say—greens rock!

➤ *CROWD IN THESE LEAFY GREENS:*
Arugula, baby greens, beet greens, collard greens, endive, kale, lettuces (all except iceberg), mustard greens, spinach, swiss chard

Low-Starch Vegetables

How low-starch veggies can make you shine: These veggies are low in natural sugars and calories while high in vitamins, minerals, phytochemicals, and antioxidants. They keep you feeling full and satiated. When you load your plate with veggies, you likely won't miss heavier foods like dairy, grains, and red meat. Eat up!

➤ *CROWD IN THESE LOW-STARCH VEGGIES:*
Artichokes, asparagus, bell peppers, broccoli, brussels sprouts, cabbage (green and red), cauliflower, celery, cucumber, eggplant, fennel, green beans, jicama, leeks, mushrooms, onions, zucchini squash (green and yellow)

Lean Proteins

How lean proteins can make you shine: Did you know your body burns more fat digesting protein than it does digesting either of the other primary macronutrients—carbohydrate and fat? Also, proteins have a complete amino acid profile to build muscle, repair tissues, and produce healthy hormones.

For the first 7 days of the reset program, stock up on our favorite lean

Did You Know Omega-3 Fatty Acids Do Your Body *Better than Good?*

Omega-3 fatty acids can help to lower triglycerides (blood fat) and boost your mood. If you're pregnant, omega-3 fatty acids can also contribute to your baby's healthy brain development.

protein—omega-3-rich fresh fish. When you can, choose wild fish over farm-raised. This is often your safest and healthiest bet because fish that are farm-raised are more likely to be contaminated with antibiotics, toxic pollutants, and chemicals that have made their way into their feed. With a little extra effort, however, you can find sustainably farmed fish that are free of antibiotics, coloring, and harmful pollutants. Sustainable and conscious fisheries continue to pop up in varied locations throughout the country. Do an online search for brands and vendors in your area that farm sustainably.

In our opinion, the best place to buy fish is from your local fish markets or natural grocers because these tend to be dedicated to sourcing local fish and often receive fresh shipments daily. Purchasing frozen fish is your next best option because it's often flash-frozen: Soon after it's caught, it's quickly brought down to -40°F to preserve its freshness. Believe it or not, frozen fish is often fresher than the fresh fish sold at the grocery store. Check the packaging; if it says "flash-frozen," you've caught a winner.

In addition to nutrient-rich fish, shop for organic free-range turkey that has been freshly roasted from a deli or your kitchen, organic free-range chicken prepared simply baked or roasted, and organic free-range eggs—the whole thing, *not* just the white. The rich and delicious yolk contains 100 percent of the egg's fat-soluble vitamins A, D, E, and K plus calcium, iron, zinc, biotin, thiamin, folate, and vitamins B_6 and B_{12}. Additionally, eggs are one of the richest dietary sources of choline, an essential micronutrient that helps cell membranes function correctly, aids nerve signaling, and transports lipids from the liver. Egg yolks also contain the carotenoids lutein and zeaxanthin, both powerful antioxidants found in brightly shaded foods that promote healthy skin and vision. Finally, numerous studies indicate that due to their high level of monosaturated fats that help lower your blood pressure, egg yolks can actually *increase* your good HDL cholesterol.

> ➤ *CROWD IN THESE LEAN PROTEINS:*
> **Canned fish like salmon, sardines, tuna (no salt or oil added), fish and shellfish (preferably wild-caught or sustainably farmed), organic chicken (skinless white meat), organic free-range eggs, organic turkey**

Healthy Fats

How healthy fats can make you shine: At 9 calories per gram, fats are the most concentrated energy source of all foods, and despite what you probably think—fats do not make you fat! Processed foods, white flour, sugar, and excess starchy carbs are behind that bulge. Healthy fats are all wonderfully lubricating to the digestive tract and beneficial to the hair, skin, and nails. Coconut oil, avocado oil, and ghee (clarified butter) will be your cooking oils for the first 7 days of the reset program. They have the highest burn temperature and may be heated without damaging their molecular structure and forming free radicals—unstable molecules that can do major damage to our healthy cells.

Coconut oil is a shelf-stable saturated fat and can tolerate heat from cooking without

Do You Know the Three Things to Consider When Selecting Fish?

1. **Is it high in omega-3 fatty acids?**

2. **Is it low in mercury and other potentially harmful substances?**

3. **Is it wild-caught or sustainably farmed?**

The following are our best picks of fish and shellfish that meet all of these favorable criteria:

Anchovies*	Mackerel*
Barramundi	Oysters
Butterfish	Pollack
Canned light tuna	Rainbow trout
Catfish	Salmon*
Cod*	Sardines*
Crab	Scallops
Flounder/sole*	Shrimp
Haddock*	Striped bass
Herring*	Sturgeon*
Lobster	Tilapia

*Highest in omega-3 fatty acids

mutating and becoming carcinogenic. Saturated fats have gotten a bad rap, but naturally occurring saturated fats are actually necessary and beneficial to the body.

Coconut oil is rich in medium-chain saturated fatty acids, which are easy for the body to break down and burn for energy versus being stored as a fat. Coconut oil can actually help boost your metabolism, and did we mention—it's absolutely delicious!

Super-smooth and buttery avocado oil will also add wonderful flavor to your food. It, too, also has a very high smoke point, making it a stellar oil for cooking at higher heat. Use avocado oil for sautéing veggies, baking fish, or any kind of roasting at higher temperatures. Whole avocados are packed with antioxidant vitamin E and minerals like potassium and magnesium; they are also a great source of fiber. They contain no starch and are predominantly composed of heart-healthy monounsaturated fats. They can deliciously replace mayonnaise, cheese, and creamy dressings.

Extra-virgin olive oil and flax oil have a lower smoke point than coconut and avocado oil, so they make excellent dressings and finishing oils. Throughout the full 28-day program, you're invited to add these nutritional and savory oils to your dishes. Extra-virgin olive oil is monounsaturated, which has been shown to help lower total cholesterol and aid in blood sugar control. It tolerates lower cooking temps, and is best for room-temperature dressings or applied in a drizzle after cooking to prevent oxidation.

Flax oil is a great source of essential omega-3 fatty acids, which most people don't get enough of, including alpha-linolenic acid. ALA can be converted into EPA and DHA, the anti-inflammatory acids commonly found in fish oil. Flax oil also promotes digestive health by lubricating the inner lining of the intestines. Flax oil is best used as a finishing oil on roasted veggies, drizzled over chilled soups, or used in salad dressings. It is extremely heat-sensitive and should not be heated.

Ghee, Did You Know?

Ghee is butter with the milk solids removed. This means you can consume it if you are lactose-intolerant because the lactose is removed with the milk solids, leaving just the oil. It's a great butter alternative because it has a high smoke point (485°F) so it will not form free radicals when heated like many vegetable oils. It also has a long shelf life and does not require refrigeration. Not to mention it has a savory nutty and buttery taste.

Store it in the fridge, preferably in a dark bottle to avoid oxidation.

> ➤ *CROWD IN THESE HEALTHY FATS:*
> **Avocado oil, coconut oil, extra-virgin olive oil, flax oil (preferably cold-pressed), ghee clarified butter**

Unsweetened Almond or Coconut Milk

How dairy-free milk can make you shine:
Non-dairy milks tend to be low in calories as well as high in vitamin E, omega-3 fatty acids, and calcium—and most grocery stores today have entire cold-case sections dedicated to them. We love both unsweetened almond and coconut milk for their high nutritional value. Almond milk is a superstar—low in calories and high in antioxidants, naturally occurring vitamin E, omega-3 fatty acids that help lower your "bad" cholesterol, and minerals like iron and calcium. In fact, almond milk is higher in calcium than cow's milk! Almond milk makes a great non-dairy alternative for tea, for cereal, or as a smoothie base.

Coconut milk is much higher in calories and natural healthy fats than almond milk, but the fats in coconut milk tend to be burned as fuel by your body rather than stored as fat. Also, the saturated fat in coconut milk, lauric acid, may actually raise your HDL "good" cholesterol levels. Coconut milk is rich in naturally occurring iron, magnesium, and zinc, and contains a small dose of B vitamins to give your metabolism and mood a boost. It's thick and creamy and makes a satisfying alternative to cow's-milk creamer in your morning coffee. Coconut milk also works wonderfully as a full-fat dairy substitute in soups, sauces, dressings and desserts.

Unroasted Nuts and Seeds

How nuts and seeds can make you shine:
Nuts and seeds are wonderful little packages of nutrients, fiber, protein, and healthy fats from nature. The fat found in nuts and seeds is predominantly monounsaturated and polyunsaturated, in the form of omega-6 fatty acids. We love our omegas, but too much omega-6 in the body can cause inflammation, which can manifest in any number of ways. So when it comes to nuts—portion control is important. We love nuts that have a nice balance of omega-3 to omega-6 fatty acids. Macadamia nuts, walnuts, chia seeds, and flaxseeds are wonderfully balanced in

this way. We also love almonds for their high vitamin E and fiber content as well as their versatility and delicious flavor. We recommend that you choose plain over roasted nuts as much as you can because the roasting process heats their oils to a high temperature that actually mutates their molecular structure into something the body cannot easily break down. Finally, always say no-no to peanuts on this program, which tend to be very difficult for the body to digest and aren't a nut anyway!

> ➤ *CROWD IN THESE UNROASTED NUTS AND SEEDS:*
> Almonds, chia seeds, flaxseeds, macadamias

Natural Sweeteners

How natural sweeteners can make you shine: Satisfy your sweet tooth without wrecking your metabolism. You will be crowding out almost all natural sweeteners on the 7-day reset while you curb your sugar cravings and reset your palate to natural sweetness. The one exception is stevia, which you will see listed as an optional ingredient in many of the juice recipes. Stevia is actually not a sugar at all. It is a plant that originated in South America and is naturally sweet. Its leaves are 300 times sweeter than regular sugar, and yet stevia has been shown not to affect blood sugar levels. While stevia is a great sugar alternative, it's important to use discretion when choosing stevia products. Look for "organic stevia" or "whole leaf stevia" on the ingredient label. Many stevia products contain added ingredients like agave that can be disruptive to your blood sugar levels and metabolism.

> ➤ *CROWD IN THESE NATURAL SWEETENERS:*
> Stevia, organic or "whole leaf"

Condiments and Vinegars

How condiments and vinegars can make you shine: They are all 5 calories or less per serving, extremely low in sugar, extremely high in flavor, and help with pH alkalization. Apple cider vinegar has a number of presumed health benefits, including weight management and pH alkalization. Balsamic is perfect if you have a sweet tooth because it has a sweeter, less acidic flavor than other vinegars. You can use it on salads, fish, meats, or roasted veggies. Dijon mustard is a dream because it brings the cream factor to dressings when whisked with a vinegar and/or healthy oil. It also makes a great dip for veggies or marinade for fish. Tamari (gluten-free soy sauce) is a salt lover's best friend because it has a deep, savory flavor that adds a salty kick to sauces, marinades, and dressing. Because it's fermented, it lacks the harmful estrogenic properties of soy and does not contain gluten as many processed soy products do. Look for reduced-sodium, non-GMO tamari.

> ➤ *CROWD IN THESE CONDIMENTS AND VINEGARS:*
> **Apple cider vinegar, balsamic vinegar, dijon mustard, non-gmo tamari (gluten-free soy sauce)**

Herbs and Spices

How herbs and spices can make you shine: Herbs and spices are the best way to flavor your food with no added calories. Without any sugar, not-so-healthy fats, carbs, preservatives, or additives, fresh herbs and spices will be your secret weapon throughout the program. Feel free to use them liberally. Have fun experimenting with a wide range of herbs and spices in the coming weeks to see how they transform your juices and meals. Many of them contain chlorophyll, antioxidants, and other vitamins and minerals that make them wonderfully beneficial to your overall health and wellness.

Salt

How salt can make you shine: Salt is an essential nutrient and electrolyte the body needs. It's also an important component of body fluids, helps to maintain blood pressure, and plays a role in brain communication with the muscles. And beyond all that—it's a wonderful flavoring for food. While the amount of processed sodium in the average American diet is too high, adding natural salt to your meals can be an important part of a healthy diet. In fact, many nutritionists agree that too little natural salt in your diet can be unhealthy. So with that, sprinkle it on, along with pepper, to any and all of your meals throughout the 28-day program.

Water

How water can make you shine: Hydration is a super important component of the Suja Juice Solution. The juices you will be drinking every day are abundant in hydration from water-dense fruits and veggies. However, you still need to load up on water. It helps to flush waste out of your system and is crucial to effective elimination. (It also helps to flush extra water weight out of your body, leaving you lighter and trimmer.) Whether you're committing only to the 7-day reset program or the full 28 days, consume extra water (filtered, preferably) in addition to the juices you're drinking in order to ensure adequate hydration and ease of elimination and water weight. Aim for three to five glasses per day or more if you're feeling it.

If plain, filtered water is hard for you to swallow or for those moments when you want a splash of something with a little more zip, try low-sodium sparkling water. In the first 7 days of the reset program, drink sparkling water with a juicy squeeze of lemon, lime, or grapefruit. Water infused with cucumber and mint leaves is also lovely. Later in the program, steep fresh fruit in a pitcher overnight, allowing it to infuse the water with added flavor. Strawberry with basil, and pineapple with lavender are both delicious and refreshing tonics. Also, feel free to steep and sip an unlimited amount of unsweetened, decaf herbal teas throughout the full 28-day program.

Elevating your health and wellness begins with cultivating an awareness and understanding of how certain foods and substances affect your physical and mental body. Now with a clear understanding of the foods you'll be crowding out over the course of the next 7 to 28 days—as well as what foods you will be crowding in for their restorative properties, which provide the healthful hydration and nourishment your body craves—you're ready to start the week that will significantly shift how you look and feel.

Q: How important is it that I use organic produce in my juice? It's expensive!

A: We believe that organic juice is the best juice you can put into your body. *Organic* means there are no chemical fertilizers, synthetic substances, irradiation, or genetically modified organisms (GMOs) used in the farming and production process of the food. Juicing makes all of the plant matter and everything it contains very easy for the body to absorb—all the nutrients, vitamins, minerals, and enzymes, and *also* any chemicals, pesticides, and potentially harmful by-products of the conventional growing environment. For this reason, we strongly believe that it's more important than ever to use organic produce in your juices.

We always encourage buying local, organic fruits and vegetables, and we understand that this expense can add up. To offset this cost, shop your local farmer's markets, where you can often find great deals on fresh organic produce because you're buying directly from the farmers. Buying in season will always be more wallet-friendly, too, because there's abundant supply available. Plus, fruits and veggies at the peak of the season are the best tasting. There's nothing better than biting into a rich and ripe,

CHAPTER 4
· · · · · · · · · ·
JUICY FAQ

sun-kissed piece of seasonal fruit. If it's not in your budget to purchase all of your produce organic, aim to purchase organic produce *for your juices*, and remind yourself that while buying organic is pricier than buying conventional, your health is your best investment.

Q: How much extra time in the kitchen will making daily juices take me?
A: You've committed to make your health and wellness a priority for the next 7 to 28 days (and we applaud you!). This level of commitment involves some extra time and effort—at least initially. Once you get into a juicy groove, it'll simply become part of your daily routine. A few tips to get you started:

- **Wash and dry** your fresh fruits and veggies as soon as you get home. As you unload your groceries, set aside your fresh produce, to rinse and scrub. Sure, this extends your grocery run a little bit longer, but it will save you time later. When it's time to juice, everything's ready to go. Save yourself even more time in the kitchen by pre-chopping carrots and celery, quartering beets, and halving lemons and cucumbers so they're juicer-ready.

- **Schedule it in.** If it takes you 15 minutes to juice and clean up, set your morning alarm so your new wake-up time is 15 minutes earlier than the night before. If you plan the time, you have the time.

- **Do the prep work.** Portion out all the ingredients for the juices you will be making for the next day and seal them in a container or a ziplock bag that you throw in the fridge. Preparing today will make your life easier tomorrow.

- **Soak overnight.** After your final juice of the day, fill up your kitchen sink with water and suds. Disassemble your juicer; throw the washable pieces like the blades, pulp receptacle, filter, and tubes into the sink; and let them soak overnight. By morning, all the pulp will have loosened up and settled to the bottom of the sink, and your juicer's pieces will only need a good wipe and rinse before you can put them back to work. (Many new juicers are dishwasher-safe, eliminating the need for hand washing, but this means running the dishwasher after every use.)

Q: What do I do with all the pulp? It feels wasteful to throw it out.

A: When juicing becomes a daily part of your life, you will indeed have a lot of pulp on your hands. Depending on the day, the Suja plant may generate thousands of pounds of pulp; we don't like to waste a good thing, either, so we recycle it. We give the majority of our left-over pulp to farmers who use it for feed and fertilizer. On a much smaller scale, you can do the same. If you have a garden, compost the scraps and add it to your soil to promote healthy growth and vitamin-rich plants. If you don't compost, bag up the pulp and give it to a friend or neighbor who does. Many schools use compost for planting children's gardens and would likely love to receive your nutrient-dense pulp. If you're a dog owner, try adding your veggie and fruit pulp into your pet food by blending it with fresh meats, flaxseeds, and sweet potato. If you're creative in the kitchen, use the pulp as an ingredient in veggie burgers (see page 174 for a tasty Bliss Burger recipe to try!). Mix the pulp with a blend of flaxseeds, nuts, herbs, and spices until a consistency is reached that holds together and tastes great. You can also throw red, orange, or green juice pulp into soups, casseroles, meat or nut loaf, sauce reductions, and baked goods like carrot and zucchini muffins to save yourself some chopping and shredding time. Your juice scraps can provide a great source of fiber and texture, along with additional flavor to some of your standard, go-to dishes.

Q: Can I make juice ahead of time? How much, and what's the best way to store it?

A: How much juice you make at one time, and how it's best to store it, absolutely depends on which type of juicer you use. If you have a centrifugal juicer, ideally you will drink your juices immediately after making them to avoid oxidation and nutrient loss which happens almost as soon as the juice is extracted. If you're making more than one serving of juice at a time, you can store it for up to 24 hours in the fridge sealed in an airtight container. Be sure you fill the container all the way to the top of the lid with juice, leaving no room for oxygen to degrade it. If you use a cold-press juicer, you may make two to three days' worth of juice at one time and use the same storage method. Juices made in both a centrifugal and a cold-press juicer can be frozen for longer periods of time to preserve the vitamins, minerals, and enzymes, and they should be frozen immediately to prevent oxidation. If you're freezing, leave about a 1-inch space at the top of the container to allow for expansion, and once you've pulled a container out of the freezer and thawed it, drink it immediately.

Q: I don't have time to juice or blend. Can I drink pre-bottled juices instead?

A: If you don't have time to make your own juices, you can shortcut this step. Because we want this program to be accessible to everyone, we've provided a compatible Juice Bar Blend for every juice in the book—a recipe that you can take to your favorite custom juice bar or juice truck to easily make for you using ingredients they will likely have on hand. These custom blends feature the same key ingredients and nutritional benefits as the comparable recipes listed throughout the program so that you can simply grab 'n' go!

Q: Do I have to drink the juices and eat the suggested meals in the exact order?

A: Week-to-week, the meal options in this program are designed to be mix-and-match within the morning, midday, and early-evening time periods, so feel free to *mix it up*. Just be sure to mix it up only within the time period and stick only to the ingredients on that week's shopping list. As far as the juices go, the order in which you consume them affects how you digest, absorb, and assimilate nutrients, so we do strongly suggest drinking each day's juices in order. Drink the lighter, water-based citrus juices in the morning on an empty stomach, as they're optimal for stimulating digestion and elimination, followed by the heavier, more complex juices at midday and in early evening. Still, while we've designed the juices and meals to follow in a specific order, we understand that everyone has a different schedule, food preferences, metabolism, and body composition. In the end, do what works best and feels right for you.

Q: Will I get enough protein on the program, especially in the first 7 days when most animal protein is crowded out?

A: Not to worry. You will be consuming as much protein as your body needs. Proteins are restorative, building-block foods and for the first 7 days of the program, you will be focusing on cleansing and resetting your body, so it's perfectly healthy and safe for you to consume less protein than you usually do.

Plus, many of the veggies and leafy greens you will be encouraged to eat more of pack a lot of protein, amino acids, and iron. Did you know that per calorie, kale has more iron than beef? This nutritional powerhouse has even been called "the new beef" because of its high iron content. One cup also contains 10 percent of the recommended daily value of omega-3 fatty acids that benefit your body in a number of ways. Hail, kale!

Q: Juices are high in sugar. I'm worried about consuming extra calories, elevating my blood sugar levels, and gaining weight.
A: Unlike white table sugar and other processed sweeteners, the juices you'll be drinking contain *natural sugars* which have a lower glycemic index than processed sugars. Has anyone ever gotten fat from eating apples? Probably not. Your body recognizes these natural sugars and utilizes them as an easily digestible source of energy for the brain and body to help you perform your daily activities and internal chemical processes. When you consume processed and refined sugars, quite the opposite happens because they are not recognizable to the body the same way fruit sugars are. Added sugars interfere with the body's internal chemistry by stimulating stress hormones and rapidly spiking blood sugar. When the body cannot easily recognize something, it isn't able to efficiently digest and metabolize it. This causes weight gain, bloating, indigestion, and skin eruptions. Consider, too, that the amount of refined, processed, and added sugar Americans typically consume in a sitting far outweighs the amount of natural sugars in the 12- to 16-ounce juices you'll be drinking throughout this program. The natural sugars in the juices have been carefully proportioned to an average adult's metabolic burn rate, and paired with whole-food meals (with protein, healthy fats, and fiber) meant to help stabilize your blood sugar rather than spike it.

Q: Can I introduce my children to these juices as I'm working through the program? Is it safe for them to consume juice regularly?
A: Fresh juice is a great vehicle for delivering nutrient- and vitamin-dense greens into your child's body that he or she may not have a strong taste for. Additionally, children are constantly burning calories to build bone and muscle tissue as well as support their high energy levels. Organic, unsweetened, natural juices

provide a steady source of natural sugar that can be efficiently used by your child's body as fuel. The sugar in organic fruits and vegetables is pure and natural and easy for their bodies to digest and metabolize, unlike processed and artificial sugars in packaged foods that are often labeled "kid-friendly" but in fact, can wreak havoc on your child's blood sugar levels.

Q: Can I do the program if I am pregnant or nursing?

A: It's best to consult with your doctor before making any dietary changes during pregnancy or post pregnancy. Many pregnant women are advised against consuming raw juices like those in this program. If your doctor advises you to skip the juices, consider following the meal plan only. The whole-food meals are nourishing to the body and provide a balance of protein, healthy fats, natural sugar, and complex carbs. For optimal health, double your portions of protein and add in a couple of additional snacks throughout the day to sustain a higher caloric intake to support you and your baby throughout your pregnancy.

Q: How many calories are in the program?

A: To give you the most feel-better health benefits (and help you drop some extra weight, as well), we've designed the combined juices + whole-food meals to come to a total of 1,200 to 1,500 calories a day. Still, calories never tell the full story—as we'll soon explain—so over the course of the program, rather than focus on the number of calories you're consuming, we encourage you to focus on the quality of the food on your plate and how it makes you feel, inside and out.

Q: Will I be hungry and have mad cravings?

A: You probably will feel some hunger in the first day or two. This is completely normal and should pass as your body acclimates to consuming fewer calories than you typically do. This does not mean, however, that you must feel hungry for the program to be effective. It's an absolute myth that if you're not starving, your body isn't cleansing itself, flushing out waste and releasing weight. After several days, expect a shift in your taste buds, a resetting of your hunger cues, and a drop in hunger levels. Also, don't be surprised if cravings for your favorite guilty pleasures diminish. It is not uncommon for people who regularly crave caffeine, sugar, grains, or a glass of wine at the end of the day to notice a significant shift in what they're hungry for. In place of many out-crowd foods, you will likely start to crave something else—nutrient-dense juice and simple, fresh foods.

Q: If I have a lot of weight to lose, can I skip the whole-food meals and drink only juice?

A: We do not recommend this. The juices you'll be drinking are predominantly carbohydrates, so it's important to incorporate whole foods into your daily menu to ensure a well-rounded intake of complex carbohydrates, lean protein, and healthy fats. These three life-supporting macronutrients work together synergistically, allowing the body to function at its best. Carbohydrates are the body and brain's main source of fuel. They're also important to the functions of the central nervous system, heart, brain, and kidneys. Proteins are the body's building blocks, aiding with tissue repair, hormone production, immune function, and preserving muscle mass. Proteins contain amino acids, some of which are essential and can only be obtained through whole foods. Natural fats are also essential for optimal health. They play an important role in vitamin absorption (the

fat-soluble vitamins A, D, E, and K cannot be absorbed without them). In addition, natural fats help cushion the organs and maintain cell membranes. If your body isn't properly fed and consistently nourished by a balanced combination of carbohydrates, protein, and natural fats, you will have a harder time metabolizing your food and shedding those unwanted pounds.

Q: Can I eat nutrition bars on the program?

A: Most "nutrition," "energy," and "protein" bars contain some combination of sugar, dried fruit, grain, soy, highly processed protein powder, synthetic vitamins, or flavorings— foods and ingredients we're encouraging you to crowd out because of the negative impact they have on your digestion and metabolism. While some options are better than others, we recommend that you avoid nutrition bars altogether for the duration of the program, whether that's for 7 days or the full 28, and focus on nutrient-dense, pure, unprocessed foods that are easy for your body to digest, assimilate, and eliminate.

Q: What do I order if I go out for a meal while I'm on the program?

A: The beauty of eating out is that you're paying to be served and satisfied, so ask for exactly what you want. You may be surprised at how willing restaurants are to fulfill your requests. You can customize pretty much every meal on a menu when you keep these solutions in mind:

- Anything can be served over a bed of greens. Swap out the pasta, rice, potatoes, or grains for a simple bed of greens.

- Anything can be made without sauce, with sauce on the side, or with a *different* sauce. When ordering a salad, ask for a vinaigrette swap or olive oil and balsamic on the side. By dressing your own salad, you control how much you consume. If you want to skip dressing altogether, but don't want to lose out on flavor, ask for a side of Dijon mustard. This condiment adds zip and zing without the calories. If you're missing the creaminess of a dairy-based dressing, add avocado, nuts, or seeds to your salad. These satisfying healthy fats will help you forget the dressing that's missing from your plate.

- Anything can be prepared in a slightly different way. It's true that most restaurants use cooking oils like soy and corn oil that can wreak havoc on your digestive system, but you are always free to request a healthier alternative—steamed instead of sautéed, baked rather than seared, poached over scrambled. Almost every restaurant has an oven, grill top, pots, and pans. For example, ask that your sautéed veggies be prepared steamed so that you avoid potentially not-so-healthy oils. Request that your pan-seared halibut be baked to skip the oil bath altogether. Order your eggs poached with salt and pepper, and savor the flavor of the rich and wholesome yolk.

Q: The first week of the program feels too restrictive to me. Can I skip ahead, or is that a fail?

A: If skipping ahead means committing to the program for any amount of time that shifts your way of eating away from not-so-healthy foods like added sugars, saturated fats, and processed foods, and toward a more nutrient-dense and balanced diet, then our answer is *yes*! That's not a fail—it's a win. The program is only a failure if you force your body to do something it doesn't want to do and you don't enjoy the process. Everyone is different, so do what feels right for you. Nobody knows your body like you do, so if crowding out whole fruits, for example, is impractical for you, skip over the first 7 days and start on day 8; if crowding out all grains feels too challenging, then skip ahead to day 15; or if you simply want to begin feeling the benefits of adding nutrient-dense juice to your existing diet, then start at day 21. The point is: Whoever you are, the Suja Juice Solution can work for you.

While the four weeks of the Suja Juice Solution build on each other, and we do recommend a full 28 days to experience the most significant shift in your health and wellness, each week has been designed to stand on its own. We've designed it this way so that wherever you are on the path to better health, you can move ahead. We understand that living a healthy lifestyle isn't always a straight path forward. There are inevitable bumps along the way, detours, and sometimes straight up dead ends. So we live by the following mantra: *Make the healthiest choices you can, and then move on.*

Q: Do I have to start all over again if I fall off the program?

A: No. One "bad" bite, meal, or day doesn't mean it's over and you're back to day one. Just start again from where you are. At your very next meal, drink the recommended juice followed by a nutritious whole-food meal. Your long-term success will be dependent on your ability to fall off the program from time to time without derailing entirely. Remind yourself that perfection isn't the goal (nor is it all that realistic). Forgive and accept yourself for being human, and then move forward in the direction of optimal health and wellness.

By prioritizing your health and wellness for the next 7 to 28 days, you've committed yourself to spend a little extra time in the kitchen, and with the right tools and a dedicated space on your countertop where you can easily throw it down, you'll find yourself getting into a juicy groove in no time. Juicing and preparing whole-food meals will simply become part of your daily routine.

A JUICER: CENTRIFUGAL VERSUS COLD-PRESSED

A juicer will soon begin to play a significant role in your new healthy lifestyle and should be selected with care. There are two types of juicers—centrifugal and cold-pressed. What's the diff? Let's start with the most common and the type you're likely most familiar with—centrifugal. A centrifugal juicer has a fast spinning blade with a mesh filter. The blade quickly shreds the produce and pushes the juice through the strainer with the force of its high spin. It's efficient, but this fast spinning motion can draw oxygen into the machine, causing the juice to oxidize, which creates nutrient loss. Additionally, micro amounts of heat are

CHAPTER 5

YOUR NEW KITCHEN TOOLS

produced by the high-power motion of the blade; this can destroy many of the heat-sensitive enzymes, vitamins, and minerals contained in the produce—the very stuff you want to start flowing into your body. Although centrifugal juices are a bit lower in nutrition than cold-pressed juices, they're still jam-packed with nutrients that are wonderful for your body, especially if consumed within 30 minutes of juicing. Our favorite brand of centrifugal juicers is Breville, which will cost you in the range of $250 to $300.

A cold-press juicer involves a grinder and a press. Your produce is slowly ground into a bag, producing zero heat and creating very little oxidation while preserving health-beneficial vitamins, enzymes, and nutrients. The bag of pulp is then pressed between two plates using extremely strong pressure that squeezes the most juice possible out of the pulp. In fact, after pressing, your pulp should be dry. This method of juicing yields a greater amount of nutrients from your fruits and veggies, and produces more juice. Another advantage of using a cold-press juicer versus a centrifugal is that you can use a smaller amount of produce and yield significantly more juice. Bonus! If you're purchasing organic produce

(and we hope you are), this savings adds up, so consider that as part of the price tag. A cold-press juicer can be expensive, but when you're juicing regularly it can quickly pay for itself. The mac daddy of all cold-press juicers is the Norwalk press, which was created by juicing pioneer Norman Walker. This is the juicer that created the first Suja juices, so naturally it holds a special place in our hearts. At $2,500 to $3,000, the Norwalk press is a major investment. The Hurom, Omega, and Breville "slow masticating" cold-press juicers are a bit more budget-friendly, do the job, and generally range in price from $300 to $500.

A BLENDER

Let's start off by clarifying that blenders are *not* juicers. A blender is a great tool for mixing liquids, but it will not extract juice from produce and leave the pulp behind. A blender will blend liquids, fruits, and veggies into smooth liquids, but the fiber and plant matter remains in the drink, making it thicker and more textured than a juice. Because of this, blended drinks require more digestive labor than juices, limiting the amount of pure juice goodness you receive into your bloodstream. If a blender is all you've got, you're still doing yourself a big favor by making the nutrients in the fruits and veggies easier to assimilate into your body, so blend away! All of the juices in this program can be made simply in your blender by adding a few key ingredients to turn them into smoothies; recipe-to-recipe, we'll show you how.

Our favorite blender is the Vitamix, because it has a very powerful blade that can tackle tough greens like kale and incorporate them into smoothies seamlessly. It can also make the smoothest, creamiest nut milks. If you don't already have a Vitamix, or if purchasing one isn't in your budget (note that you can often find great deals on new or refurbished machines on Amazon, eBay, and Craigslist), any good blender with a powerful blade will do. Typically, the higher the speeds, the more powerful the blade. Before you buy, browse online reviews to determine what model will achieve your blending goals. Some blenders will be better at making simple soups than at tackling greens. Ask your kitchen store if they'll allow you to test drive before purchase. Many will, and are already set up for demonstrations.

A FOOD PROCESSOR

A food processor is just what it sounds like—a processor for food. These machines can save you valuable time and arm labor. Plus, they're relatively cheap. For 40 bucks or so, you can arm yourself with a more-than-capable machine. For recipes calling for chopped herbs, grated ginger, or minced garlic, simply toss the ingredients into your food processor and hit CHOP. A food processor can also be used to easily make guacamole, salsa, salad dressing, hummus, and nut butters in almost no time at all. Making your own dips, dressings, and butters can significantly lower your grocery store costs and allows you to use fresh, organic ingredients, bypassing the less-than-healthy versions packaged and bottled on the shelves.

TOOLS AND GADGETS

Dehydrator
Cooking food destroys a fair amount of enzymes, vitamins, antioxidants, and minerals, so incorporating raw foods into your

diet can give you some of those valuable nutrients back. Did you know that by simply swapping one cooked food for its raw version at every meal, you can boost the nutritional benefits by up to 50 percent? Now, if you're not too excited to add a serving of raw veggies to your plate, get this—the standard definition of *raw foods* is "foods that have not been heated above 118°F." Meaning, you can still cook your raw food. This is where a dehydrator comes in handy. A dehydrator is essentially a mini oven that can be set to very low temperatures. At 115°F, you can safely bake kale chips, seasoned nuts, flax crackers, veggie burgers, and veggie chips without "cooking out" their nutrients. While it's not an essential kitchen tool, a dehydrator can make a fun and tasty addition to this program.

Nut Milk Bag

The secret to smooth and silky nut milks is the nut milk bag. This is a mesh bag that works like a strainer. Pour your blended nut-and-water mixture through your nut milk bag to remove all the gritty nut pulp, leaving only creamy milk behind. You can find these bags online; choose one in a natural fiber like cotton, hemp, or linen. As an alternative method, try using organic cheesecloth to strain juice over a mesh strainer.

6-Inch Standard Chef Knife

You don't have to be a chef to own one of these. Really, this knife should be renamed "the novice's knife" because if you do *any* amount of cooking or food prep, you should have one. It does it all—chopping, dicing, mincing, and cubing just about anything.

Cutting Board

Think of your cutting board as your personal workspace. It's where you can do all your prep work and experiment with different ways of slicing and dicing without making the kind of mess you don't want to clean up. Plastic cutting boards are cheap and easy to clean, but we suggest investing in wood. A wooden cutting board is gentler on your knives, better for the environment, and considered safer because it doesn't leach potentially harmful chemicals into your food. There's been some public debate on whether or not wooden boards harbor germs more than plastic, but various studies indicate that bacteria may actually become trapped in the grain of the wood, where they die. Either way, if you invest in plastic or wood, routine cleaning with soap and water is important to effectively safeguard against bacteria and germs.

Mason Jars

We recommend storing your juice in glass rather than plastic containers, and mason jars are our favorite. They're super trendy right now; you can find them in stores like Target, Costco, and Walmart. When you chill your juice in the fridge, be sure to fill the jar all the way to the top to cut down on oxidation and nutrient loss. When you're freezing glass containers, leave a little room at the top or the glass will likely crack when the juice freezes.

Spiralizer

This is a fun gadget that can make creative food art out of almost any fruit or veggie you can buy. Make zucchini ribbons to replace the grains in a bowl of pasta marinara. Bake swirly and savory sweet potato fries to satisfy your craving for white potatoes. Decorate your salads with carrot and beet spirals. A spiralizer allows you to get artsy with the presentation of your meals.

1-Quart Glass Measuring Cup

Even though all juice recipes throughout the program have been carefully measured, juice yields tend to vary so by placing a measuring cup under the spout of your juicer, you can easily measure the desired quantity of your juice. This method comes in handy when you want to juice or blend larger quantities that you set aside or freeze for later.

PART 2

The
SUJA JUICE SOLUTION

BEFORE THE PROGRAM

The Suja Juice Solution is a hydration- and whole-food-centered plan created to give you the nutrition your body needs through wholesome, organic fruits and vegetables, healthy fats, and lean proteins. Daily, you will consume three delicious juices that provide your body with healthful hydration and vitamins, minerals, and beneficial antioxidants. In addition, you will consume three whole-food meals. Together, the juices and meals provide your body with a complete range of plant-based nutrition. While the Suja Juice Solution is a gentle program that your body will love, unless you already eat this way, it will take some getting used to. For this reason, we recommend that you ease into the program by giving yourself a revving jump start.

One to three days before you jump into the reset program, give yourself a gentle jump start by taking the following steps:

- Consider lightening up on out-crowd foods (see chapter 3 for a full list).

- Hydrate.

CHAPTER 6

GIVE YOURSELF a REVVING JUMP START

- Move your body.

- Set up your kitchen.

- Join a community.

BEGIN TO CROWD OUT FOODS

Lighten up on your intake of out-crowd foods: processed foods, sugar, white flour and whole grains, dairy, caffeine, alcohol, red meat, and artificial ingredients like preservatives, high-fructose corn syrup, and hydrogenated fats. In the meantime, dial up your intake of whole, fresh fruits, veggies, lean protein, and healthy fats to give your body a jump start for the first 7 days of the reset program. By giving yourself a few days to get with the program, so to speak, you help your body ease into a new way of nourishing yourself with fresh, clean, and pure foods. Reducing some of the most difficult-to-digest and addictive foods in your diet a few days before you remove them entirely will make the transition to the program less of a shock, or a challenge.

If you drink caffeine, this jump-start phase can help minimize the withdrawal effect. Try cutting your intake of caffeine down by 25 percent on day 1; 50 percent by day 2; and 75 percent by day 3. Or if you're able, make the switch to decaf tea or coffee in one single go (both still have trace amounts of caffeine). By gradually crowding out caffeine, you're less likely to suffer from withdrawal once you start the program.

Also, what you probably don't know is that the green juices you'll be drinking in the first 7 days of the reset program are the best way to stop a caffeine addiction dead in its tracks. The rich chlorophyll content of leafy greens oxygenates the blood, making you feel alert and focused. After a few days of drinking fresh, delicious hydrating green juices, caffeinated tea, coffee, and soda will likely taste acidic and unappealing.

HYDRATE

Hydration is one of our favorite words, and it is a key component of the Suja Juice Solution. As you prepare for the first 7 days of the reset program, hydrate with still water (filtered, preferably), sparkling water, or decaffeinated herbal tea. Water helps to flush waste and extra water weight out of your system and is crucial to effective detoxification. Begin to get in the habit of drinking three to five glasses per day to ensure adequate hydration and ease of elimination.

KEEP MOVING

For the next one to three days, continue your regular exercise routine. Are you a runner? Keep up the pace. Do you surf, bike, swim, or hike? Maintain the intensity. By continuing to exercise and work out as you normally do at the same time you begin to crowd out not-so-healthy foods, you actually rev up the detoxification process as you head into week 1 of the program.

SET UP YOUR KITCHEN

Refer back to chapter 5, *Your New Kitchen Tools*, to be sure you have all the necessary tools on hand to begin juicing and preparing fresh whole-food meals with ease. We also suggest that you do your grocery shopping before the start of the program. Take a look at the juices and whole-food mini meal recipes for the first 7 days of the program and purchase all the fresh ingredients you will need (see chapter 7 shopping list). We've made shopping easy for you by including a comprehensive shopping list for each week of the program.

Shopping ahead will save you frantic, frustrating runs to the store, and the temptation to eat whatever you can get your hands on. If your grocery store or natural market doesn't carry everything you will need (dandelion greens aren't always easy to find, after all), take the next few days to locate the store or stores that do.

Finally, take stock of your kitchen pantry and throw out, or give away, anything that isn't on your week 1 shopping list. The crackers, popcorn, peanut butter jars, and chocolate bars have got to go! Out of sight may not be completely out of mind, but soon after you remove these out-crowd foods and focus on fresh vegetables, fruits, and healthy fats instead, you may forget they were ever there.

CREATE A COMMUNITY

You're more likely to stick with the program if you enlist friends, family members, or colleagues to join you. Is there someone in your life who's similarly interested in feeling and looking better and willing to commit to shifting a few not-so-healthy habits to get there? Invite them to join you on your health and wellness journey, at least for the initial 7 days. Maybe you have a group of friends or office-mates who want to reset their bodies to a cleaner, more balanced state. Seek out peeps who share your health and wellness goals and with whom you can connect regularly throughout the program. If you are interested in continuing your journey through inspiration and encouragement, join the free digital community we've created on www.sujajuice.com/The-Suja-Juice-Solution. There you can join with others following the program and gain access to bonus material including recipes and health and wellness tips. There is also space for you to interface with your peers and add your insights and experiences to the conversation. By coming together and sharing our weak moments, triumphs, frustrations, and fears, we learn from and support each other along the way toward a healthier lifestyle.

Fewer sugar cravings and less water retention. Heightened focus and more energy. Sounds pretty good, doesn't it? Over the course of the next week, you will begin to feel and look better than you do today by taking two simple steps:

Step 1. Add three nutrient-dense juices every day.

Step 2. Crowd out not-so-healthy foods with vitamin-rich healthier foods.

HOW DO I DO THIS?

Starting today, you will drink three glasses of organic, nutrient-dense, high-quality juice that you either prepare at home or grab 'n' go from your local juice bar. Fueled by the power of enzymes, chlorophyll, and concentrated clean, green, and vibrant nutrition, these juices will provide you with the healthful hydration, vitamins, minerals, and nourishment your body needs and truly craves, while also enabling your body to efficiently hydrate and flush out waste and release weight. Best of all, these juices are delicious: Our recipes

WEEK 1: 7 DAYS to RESET
1 week, 2 steps, 3 juices

are inspired by taste profiles from around the world.

In addition to drinking vegetable and fruit juices in the morning, at midday, and in the early evening, you will enjoy three supplemental whole-food meals that complement the colorful flavor of the juices you're drinking and also create a harmonious synergy with the hydration, vital nutrients, amino acids, omega-3 fatty acids, and antioxidants they provide. Together, the high-powered juices and whole-food meals provide your body with a complete and balanced range of plant-based nutrition with lean protein, healthy fats, and complex carbohydrates.

We believe that choices make life interesting—and meals so much more appetizing and fun to eat—so this week is front-loaded with a beautiful array of nutrient-dense juices packed with a variety of low-glycemic fruits and veggies, along with whole-food options to choose from that are easy to shop for and prepare. These original recipes were carefully crafted by head of innovation for Suja Bryan Riblett and certified holistic health coach and nutritional counselor Annie Lawless, and they will become the starter, or "base plate," from which all other recipes throughout the 28-day program are built, becoming more complex and substantial as the weeks progress. This means that once you learn how to master this first batch of recipes—and they're all relatively simple to throw together—it just becomes a matter of adding more and more delicious and nutrient-dense ingredients to them! If, however, you're someone who craves more variety or likes to experiment in the kitchen, you're invited to create your own culinary adventures instead from the list of ingredients on this week's shopping list.

This week your juice and whole-food meals are created from gentle and easily digestible in-crowd foods like leafy greens, low-glycemic veggies, lean proteins, and the healthiest fats. When you consume gentle foods, your digestive system doesn't have to work so hard. It can rest, reset, and focus its attention on releasing waste and excess weight.

Your Week 1: Reset Meal Plan at a Glance

MORNING JUICE

Sweet and Simple *or* Spa Kick

MORNING MEAL

Charged-Up Chia Pudding *or* Under the Sea Spinach Omelet *or* Sunrise Grapefruit and Avocado Salad

MIDDAY JUICE

Leafy Grapefruit Kick *or* Fennel and Friends

MIDDAY MEAL

Lentil Love Salad *or* Avocado Tuna Collard Roll *or* Kale-ifornia Salad

EARLY-EVENING JUICE

Leafy Grapefruit Kick *or* Fennel and Friends

EARLY-EVENING MEAL

Simply Salmon *or* Zesty Zucchini Basil Soup *or* Totally Guacamoly Tacos

EAT MORE OF THESE IN-CROWD FOODS

For the next 7 days, crowd in the following "in-crowd" foods:

Leafy greens: Arugula, baby greens, beet greens, collard greens, endive, kale, all lettuce (except iceberg), mustard greens, spinach, Swiss chard

Low-starch veggies: Artichoke, asparagus, bell peppers, broccoli, Brussels sprouts, cabbage (green and red), cauliflower, celery, cucumber, eggplant, fennel, green beans, jicama, leeks, mushrooms, onions, zucchini squash (green and yellow)

Legumes: Lentils only

Non-dairy milk: Unsweetened almond milk, unsweetened coconut milk

Whole fruit: Avocado, grapefruit, lemon, lime, tomato (oranges allowed in the soup recipe only)

Lean proteins: Fish and shellfish (preferably wild-caught or sustainably farmed), canned fish like salmon, sardines, and tuna (no salt or oil added), organic turkey, organic chicken (skinless white meat), organic free-range whole eggs

Good fats: Avocado oil, coconut oil, cold-pressed flax oil, extra-virgin olive oil, ghee (clarified butter)

Unroasted nuts and seeds: Almonds, macadamias, and walnuts; chia seeds and flaxseeds

Condiments: Apple cider vinegar, balsamic vinegar, Dijon mustard, non-GMO tamari (gluten-free soy sauce)

Herbs and spices: All

Natural Sweeteners: Coconut water (unsweetened), stevia (organic or "whole leaf"

EAT LESS OF THESE OUT-CROWD FOODS

The Suja Juice Solution is a hydration- and whole-food-centered plan created to eliminate anything that slows you down and holds you back from feeling and looking your best.

Throughout the next 7 days, we strongly suggest crowding out the following foods and ingredients so you can crowd in more of the feel-your-best stuff:

Grains: All, including gluten-free

Legumes: All except lentils, including peanuts

Higher-starch veggies: Beets, carrots, corn, green garden peas, pumpkin, sugar snap peas, sweet potatoes, white potatoes, winter squash (acorn, butternut, delicata, Hubbard, kabocha, pumpkin, spaghetti), yams

Refined and non-fruit sugar: Agave, all artificial sweeteners, beet sugar, brown rice syrup, brown sugar, coconut sugar, corn syrup, date sugar, evaporated cane juice, honey, jellies and jams, lactose, maple syrup, molasses, "raw" sugar, refined white sugar, Sucanat, turbinado sugar (stevia is the exception)

Whole fruits: All except avocado, lemon, lime, grapefruit, tomato

Dried fruits: All

Red meat: Bacon, beef, bison, duck, game meats, lamb, pork, rabbit, sausage (all)

Lunch meat: All

Dairy: All

Bad fats: Canola oil, corn oil, cottonseed oil, grapeseed oil, hydrogenated or partially hydrogenated oil, margarine, peanut oil, rice bran oil, safflower oil, soybean oil, sunflower oil

Soy products: Edamame, soybean oil, soy cheese, soy meats, soy milk, soy protein powder, soy yogurt, tempeh, tofu

Processed and packaged foods

Caffeine

Alcohol

Nutrition Is the Best Ammunition!

If you haven't already, consider crowding out, and even *throwing out*, many of these foods and ingredients from your fridge and kitchen pantry. This doesn't mean you'll never enjoy them again, so if you're feeling panicky that you won't ever have another hot morning cup of coffee, relax. As soon as next week, you'll be invited to reintroduce many of the foods above, and yes, a little caffeine is one of them. But for the purposes of flushing out waste, cleansing your system, and resetting your body to a more balanced state, we encourage you to remove them from your plate for the next 7 days.

The nutrients in high-powered fruit and vegetable juice and whole-food goodness is what your body needs in order to function optimally. When you give your body what it truly desires, it no longer holds on to what it doesn't. Given the opportunity, your body will quickly and relatively easily reset itself to a healthier, more vibrant state, *even in just 7 days*.

CALORIES DON'T TELL THE WHOLE STORY

To experience the most feel-better, health benefits this week, portion control is something to pay attention to, but because we believe that your focus should be on quality over quantity, we want to assure you right now that the combined juices + whole-food mini meals don't exceed a total of 1,200 to

1,500 calories a day. In other words, we've already done the calorie counting for you. You're welcome.

If counting calories is something you've always done, and if you believe you need to keep your calories in close check in order to drop bad habits and excess fat, this new lifestyle shift may feel difficult for you. Try to let go. For the next 7 days, rather than focusing on a magic number, try shifting your attention toward the *quality* of your food over the quantity.

It may surprise you to learn that higher-quality food is often higher in calories. More surprising, maybe, is that more calories don't necessarily lead to weight gain. Yep, it's true. Would you believe that your average candy bar weighs in at 250 calories where one medium avocado rounds up to 350? The chocolate bar has significantly fewer calories, but the avocado is still the better choice because its natural monosaturated fat is so much better for you. (This type of fat raises your levels of good HDL cholesterol and lowers triglycerides without raising bad LDL cholesterol levels.) Not only does your body benefit more from an avocado that is higher in calories and fat, but also it can be metabolized much more efficiently

This Could Totally Be You:
7 Days to Forever

"Juice satiates my desire for all-things-sweet because of how quenching and satisfying it is. I now have a juice every morning to not only kick-start my metabolism, but to kick-start my day. I swear I wouldn't feel ready for those early appointments or meetings without that first-thing juice! I honestly can't remember my existence before juicing. It's changed my life; for the better, and for the more fruitful."

—Nicole Moriarty, 33, grateful yogi

This Could Totally Be You:
Juice Changed My Taste for Everything

"I started drinking juice about 2 years ago. I was overweight, very sluggish, had little energy, was bloated, irregular and just not happy. I used to eat donuts, chips—anything salty and sweet. I also enjoyed my cocktails. I decided I needed to change something. I went on a 5-day juice cleanse and noticed a difference after day 2. I felt energized when I woke up, and was feeling less bloated. By the fifth day, I'd lost five pounds and felt terrific. It was the motivation I needed to start eating clean. I now juice regularly and it helps curb my cravings for sweets and salty foods—I actually crave greens! I've also noticed that my nails are thicker and stronger and I believe it helps me with PMS symptoms. Now my entire family eats healthy, too. We skip fast food and plan ahead. I work out almost every day and only enjoy cocktails at special events. I'm inspired to be healthy, and to live a better life."

—Kelly Frankfather, 37, mother, gardener, and small business owner

than foods that are highly processed and full of refined sugars. When you eat food that your body cannot easily digest, assimilate, and eliminate, it stores it as fat. Think of it this way: Waste = weight.

The calorie count of any food you eat is irrelevant because it's how your body burns those calories as fuel that matters most. Eating "100-calorie," "low-calorie," "low-carb," "fat-free," or "diet" foods will often lead to weight gain faster than eating a high-calorie diet rich in complex carbs and natural fats, because your body cannot efficiently metabolize them. Calories never tell the full story, so get your mind off the number and focus instead on eating high-quality foods that make your body sing versus low-quality empty calories that slow your body down.

WEEK 1 MEAL PLAN

Each day this week, you will *follow the same juice + meal plan for morning, midday, and early evening*.

Morning

Start your day on an empty stomach, and rehydrate with an invigorating citrus juice. By drinking your morning juice on an empty stomach, you allow your body to use and metabolize the nutrients quickly and efficiently without getting hung up by proteins, fats, or fiber from any food that you consumed prior. Lemon, lime, and grapefruit juice are perfect detoxifying tonics first thing in the morning because these citrusy fruits stimulate your body's natural enzymes and kick your metabolism into gear. Also, the juice of just one lemon gives you a third of your daily vitamin C intake, along with a

Custom Blends

If you're short on time in the kitchen, order a custom blend at your local juice bar or juice truck. We've simplified all of the juice recipes in the program to Juice Bar Blends, so you can grab 'n' go. For blender users, we've made each recipe blender-friendly by adding a few key ingredients that will turn it into a smoothie (see chapter 12).

strong dose of potassium and calcium. Lemons, limes, and grapefruits are extremely low in sugar, which makes them great for flavoring juice without adding calories, and for promoting healthy blood sugar.

MORNING JUICE

Sweet and Simple, page 135

Spa Kick, page 135

Thirty minutes later, or when hunger appears, you will eat your morning meal (see chapter 12). Your first whole-food meal of the day should be hydrating and light. Your digestive tract has been resting overnight, so you don't want to jolt it awake immediately. You want to slowly ease it back into operation, but by all means—eat! Mornings can be rushed and hectic, and yet carving out some time to take care of yourself and nourish your body first thing will help you to feel energetic and satisfied throughout the day, and over the course of the next 7 days.

MORNING MEAL

Charged-Up Chia Pudding, page 136

Under the Sea Spinach Omelet, page 137

Sunrise Grapefruit and Avocado Salad, page 137

We've created three morning meal recipes for you to choose from this week. You can eat them in whatever order you desire (eat the same thing every morning if you wish).

If you crave more variety, you're invited to create your own morning meal by combining 4 ounces lean protein, unlimited fresh green veggies, and 1 tablespoon healthy oil *or* 2 tablespoons nuts *or* ⅓ avocado. For vegetarians, combine ¾ cup cooked lentils, unlimited fresh green veggies, and 1 tablespoon healthy oil *or* 2 tablespoons nuts *or* ⅓ avocado.

Midday

At midday when you feel the need for something, enjoy a 16-ounce green juice (recipes on pages 138–139). These midday and early-evening juices are packed with mild, refreshing greens that will soothe your tummy and provide you with an alkaline rush of pure leafy green goodness. A kick of citrus will help continue to boost your metabolism and promote healthy blood sugar while the hint of mint and ginger aid in digestion. Another superstar ingredient in these juices is parsley, a powerful herbal source of vitamin C, and kale, one of the most nutrient-dense vegetables on the planet, is jam-packed with vitamins K, A, and C, along with iron and folic acid.

MIDDAY JUICE

Leafy Grapefruit Kick, page 138

Fennel and Friends, page 139

If you feel satisfied after your midday juice—and don't be surprised if you do—wait until you feel hungry again before you eat your midday meal (see chapter 12). It's important to eat only when you're truly hungry, and allow your body to fully digest before consuming your next meal.

MIDDAY MEAL

Lentil Love Salad, page 139

Avocado Tuna Collard Roll, page 140

Kale-ifornia Salad, page 140

Prepare any of the three recipes provided, or create your own midday meal by combining 4 ounces lean protein, unlimited fresh green veggies, and 1 tablespoon healthy oil *or* 2 tablespoons nuts *or* ⅓ avocado. For vegetarians, combine ¾ cup cooked lentils, unlimited fresh green veggies, and 1 tablespoon healthy oil *or* 2 tablespoons nuts *or* ⅓ avocado.

Keep in mind that when you're on the go and you need to eat and run, it's easier to stick to the program if you plan ahead. Stash portable in-crowd foods in your purse, car, desk drawer, or office fridge—avocados, canned tuna, raw nuts, and small packets of your favorite condiments like stevia, Dijon mustard, sea salt, cinnamon, or garlic. When you have a few healthy ingredients on hand, you can easily assemble a meal even in a pinch.

Juice Prep

When you're preparing your midday green juice, double the recipe (32 ounces) to generate enough for both your afternoon and evening hydration. Remember, you can make your juices ahead of time if that makes life easier. If you're making more than one serving of juice at a time using a centrifugal juicer, you can store it for up to 24 hours in the fridge sealed in an airtight container. Be sure you fill the container all the way to the top of the lid with juice, leaving no room for oxygen to degrade it. If you use a cold-press juicer, you may make three to four days' worth of juice at one time; use the same storage method. If you're freezing, leave a 1-inch space at the top of the container to allow for expansion. Once you've pulled it out of the freezer and thawed it, drink it immediately.

Early Evening

In late afternoon or early evening when you start to feel hungry again, drink the remaining 16 ounces of the green juice you prepared at midday.

EARLY-EVENING JUICE

Leafy Grapefruit Kick, page 138

Fennel and Friends, page 139

Thirty minutes later, or when hunger reappears, prepare your early-evening mini meal (see chapter 12). Again, choose to prepare any of the three recipes provided, or create your own evening meal by combining 4 ounces lean protein, unlimited fresh green veggies, and 1 tablespoon healthy oil *or* 2 tablespoons nuts *or* ⅓ avocado. For vegetarians, combine ¾ cup cooked lentils, unlimited fresh green veggies, and 1 tablespoon healthy oil *or* 2 tablespoons nuts *or* ⅓ avocado. Consume this final whole-food meal of the day a minimum of two to three hours before bed to allow your body to fully digest *before* sleep. When you're sleeping, your body pushes the PAUSE button on digestion so it can focus on other important functions like cleansing and removing waste.

EARLY-EVENING MINI MEAL

Simply Salmon, page 141

Zesty Zucchini Basil Soup, page 141

Totally Guacamoly Tacos, page 142

WELLNESS CHECK: NEED A PICK-ME-UP?

If you find yourself battling with cravings and low energy this week, know that this is normal. In fact, you probably will feel some amount of food lust and fatigue in the first day or two of the program. You're likely to be consuming fewer calories than you're used to, and your body is acclimating to digesting more liquids than solid food. Still, take a minute and check in. Often the sensation of hunger we feel is not true physical hunger; rather, it's the ritual and comfort of eating what we crave. Instead of opening the fridge, consider what else might lift and fill you up right now. Other than food, what satisfies and feeds you? Are you a painter? Pick up a paintbrush. If you read, pick up a book. If you write, pick up a pen. If you garden, pick up a shovel. If you like to gab, pick up the phone and call a good friend.

WEEK 1 MOVE YOUR BODY: LIGHT EXERCISE

Perform light exercise, like leisurely walking, deep breathing and stretching, or restorative yoga for 15 to 30 minutes a day.

Physical activity is a wonderful way to reset your body this week; movement releases chemicals to the brain such as serotonin that make you feel happy and energized. It also stimulates the lymphatic system, respiration, and perspiration—all key components of digestion and elimination. Take advantage of gentle forms of exercise like restorative yoga where many of the poses help stimulate digestion and elimination of wastes by massaging the organs, reversing blood flow, and increasing circulation. Stretching and walking also promote the circulation of blood, and the slow contraction of muscles aids in digestion and cleansing. If you're usually very active, give yourself permission this week to take a physical time-out (you deserve it!), and give your body a chance to reset and restore. As you progress through the full 28-day program, your physical activity will intensify and ramp back up to match the quantity of food you're eating, but this week you're eating less, so physically exerting yourself less is what your body needs. At the end of the full 28-day program, you will return to your normal exercise routine fully rejuvenated and reenergized.

SOAK AND SLEEP

Throughout the first 7 days of the Suja Juice Solution, it's so important to be gentle with yourself as you shift many of your not-so-healthy habits. Even when done gradually and gently, change can be a source of anxiety and stress on your physical and mental body, so in addition to focusing on light movement and deep-breathing exercises that don't place heavy demands on your physical body, consider treating yourself to a massage to further promote circulation of the lymphatic system and expedite the release of metabolic waste from your body. Your skin is your largest elimination organ, so even just 10 minutes in your spa or gym's steam room can help to release toxic buildup. A hot Epsom salt bath at home can also stimulate circulation and help your body reset to a cleaner, more balanced state.

Finally, get plenty of rest this week. You may notice that you're a little more fatigued than usual. Again, this is because you're eating less and also because your body is hard at work cleaning house! Sleep is important throughout the full 28-day program, but especially during these first 7 days when your body is resetting itself. It's when you're sleeping that your body rebuilds and repairs, so get plenty of rest and know that you will soon be feeling lighter, brighter, and better than you did just one week ago.

WEEK 1 SHOPPING LIST

Your Week 1 shopping list includes all the ingredients you'll need over the course of the next 7 days to create a powerhouse pantry and fresh-stocked fridge. You can create all the reset week juices and recipes plus 7 days of create-your-own nutritious and delicious dishes from this simple list of ingredients. It's all about getting creative!

This Could Totally Be You:
Juice Helps Me Feel Healthier!

"Since incorporating juice into my lifestyle and new diet, I've seen a huge difference healthwise. I used to be addicted to candy and sugary treats. Now my cravings have drastically subsided. When they do hit, I grab a juice. If I'm craving coffee—my go-to is juice. I can enjoy it guilt-free! Also, I don't worry about taking vitamins anymore because I drink them instead! How I feel in my body has drastically changed along with my new love of juicing."

—Jillian McCarthy, 23, hiker, yoga and barre enthusiast

Fresh Produce

Artichoke	Fennel
Arugula	Green beans
Asparagus	Green leaf lettuce
Baby greens	Green onion
Bean sprouts	Jicama
Beet greens	Kale (Jacinto)
Bell pepper	Leeks
Bok choy	Mushrooms
Broccoli	Mustard greens
Brussels sprouts	Pea sprouts
Butter lettuce	Red onion
Cabbage (green and red)	Romaine leaf lettuce
Cauliflower	Shallots
Celery	Spinach
Collard greens	Swiss chard
Cucumber	Watercress
Dandelion greens	Zucchini (green and yellow)
Eggplant	
Endive	

Fresh Whole Fruit

Avocados	Oranges (in soup only)
Grapefruit	Tomatoes (any)
Lemons	
Limes	

Week 1 Shopping Tip: Farmer's Markets

If you've never been to a farmer's market, it's time to get going! Your local farmer's market is your source for fresh, vibrant, seasonal, organic, and flavorful produce—and often at lower prices than your natural food grocer. Consider hitting your local farmer's market (they are usually held on a Saturday or Sunday) with your shopping list in hand before heading to the supermarket or your natural foods grocer. Stock up on everything you can. Not only can this save you money, but you're often buying from the farmer who actually grew your food and who can tell you everything you need to know about how it was grown and harvested. A farmer's market is also a great place to become familiar with what produce is in season in the area you live, and to broaden your exposure to a wider variety of fruits and veggies.

Proteins

Canned salmon, sardines, or tuna (no oil or sodium)

Chicken (organic, skinless, white meat)

Eggs (organic, free-range)

Lentils

Turkey (organic, oven-roasted)

Wild-caught fish, shellfish (see page 31 for a list of the healthiest and safest choices)

Healthy Fats: Nuts and Seeds

(Preferably unroasted, unsalted)

Almonds

Chia seeds

Flaxseeds

Macadamia nuts

Walnuts

Fresh and Dried Herbs

Any and all! This week prepare juices and whole-food with your favorite dried or fresh herbs

This Could Totally Be You:
Juice Calmed My Unhealthy Cravings

"I drank way too much coffee, was addicted to sugar and could stand to lose some weight. I supplemented the same food I would otherwise eat with fresh juices and within days, I could feel and see my body responding to the juice—for the first time in my life my skin started to clear. My wife actually said it was 'smooth'—something I'd never heard her say before. Also, I was drinking less coffee. I just wasn't craving it. And, I was sleeping better. A month later, my cravings for sugar were practically gone, I was snacking less throughout the day and my weight was down. I was hooked!"

—James Brennan, co-founder of Suja Juice

Spices and Seasonings

Any and all! This week prepare juices and whole food with your favorite dried or fresh spices and seasonings

Non-dairy milk

Almond milk
(unsweetened)

Coconut milk
(unsweetened)

Natural Sweeteners

Coconut water
(unsweetened)

Stevia (organic or
"whole leaf")

Shredded coconut
(unsweetened)

Essential Oils and Pantry Staples

Apple cider
vinegar

Decaffeinated
herbal tea

Avocado oil

Dijon mustard

Balsamic vinegar

Extra-virgin
olive oil

Broth, vegetable
and chicken (low
sodium, no yeast
or sugar)

Ghee (clarified
butter)

Tamari (gluten-
free soy sauce)

Coconut oil

Vinegar

Cold-pressed
flax oil

After completing the 7-day reset program, you will likely experience fewer sugar cravings and less water retention. You may also be noticing heightened focus and more energy. These are the inevitable (and awesome!) results of crowding out not-so-healthy habits and crowding in a combination of concentrated clean, green, and vibrant nutrition in the form of fresh juices and wholesome foods. You're giving your body what it truly needs and craves, while also enabling it to efficiently hydrate and flush out released waste and weight. It feels good, doesn't it—to let go of what your body doesn't need, or want, so that a more radiant you can shine through? Continue with the program for another 7 days and you'll begin to understand what it really means to glow!

How do you feel? Leaner, lighter, and brighter? More balanced and mentally focused? Have the morning citrus juices and invigorating midday greens begun to replace your taste for zany-brain caffeine? There's a reason that nutrient-dense green juice is the best way to stop a mad caffeine addiction dead in its tracks: The chlorophyll content of leafy greens oxygenates the blood, making you feel alert and focused. You may also have noticed over the past week that your craving for sugar has decreased, and in its place is a new appreciation for the natural sweetness and subtle flavors in the juices and dishes you're preparing. With your body and mind reset to a healthier equilibrium, what do you say to keepin' the good feelings going? If you feel good now, imagine how you'll feel after another 7 days!

As mentioned earlier, the Suja Juice Solution was created both for people who want a quick and powerful 7-day reset, and for those who prefer to continue with a longer maintenance plan. Of course what you do is totally up to you, but if we had it our way, you'd continue with the program for maximum benefits and results, and also to ease your body

CHAPTER 8

WEEK 2: 7 DAYS to REINFORCE

1 week, 2 steps, 3 juices

back into operation without shocking and confusing it. By reinforcing clean nutrition for another 7 days and gradually reintroducing foods back onto your plate, you give your body a chance to catch up while continuing the important cleansing process.

Your Week 2: Reinforce Meal Plan at a Glance

MORNING JUICE

Beet You to the Top *or* **Balance**

MORNING MEAL

Apple Pie That You Can't Buy *or* **Sweet Potato Perfection** *or* **Surfer's Delight**

MIDDAY JUICE

Crimson Berry *or* **Life Line**

MIDDAY MEAL

Roasted Ruby Salad *or* **San Diego Sando** *or* **Hot Bod Hummus Plate**

EARLY-EVENING JUICE

Crimson Berry *or* **Life Line**

EARLY-EVENING MEAL

Heavenly Halibut and Garlicky Greens *or* **Liquid Sunshine** *or* **Kale-ifornia Salad 2.0**

HOW DO I DO THIS?

It's simple. The next 7 days will look very similar to the first week of the program. You will:

Step 1. Add three juices every day.

Step 2. Continue to crowd out not-so-healthy foods.

The only significant difference this week is that you will add back onto your plate many complex carbohydrates that were on the out-crowd list last week. Hurray! Also, your juice options double and your meals become a bit more substantial with an additional 100 to 200 calories added to the morning, midday, and early-evening recipes (not that you're counting calories!).

Additionally this week, you're allowed a midday snack. If you find yourself hungry between morning and midday, we strongly recommend that you eat. Snacking is not cheating. If you're truly hungry, you need to eat! By ignoring your body's true hunger cues and allowing yourself to get too hungry, you set yourself up for overeating not-so-healthy foods. At some point your hunger wins, and this is when you find yourself

This Could Totally Be You:
More Energy and Focus

"I started drinking organic, natural juices when I was a freshman at the University of San Diego. Juice quickly became my 'gateway drug' from a conventional and not-so-healthy lifestyle to a more conscious and healthy one. Once I started drinking juice, I immediately noticed my appetite shifted and that changed how I shopped for groceries and what I ultimately ate. I dropped the occasional energy drink and had no craving for the dorm room junk food. Organic juices and fresh food tasted so much better to me. Plus, the juice I was drinking was giving me more energy to concentrate on coursework and be physically active. I was going to class, working 40 hour weeks and still found energy to hit Pilates six days a week. I knew there was no way I was going back to my old eating habits. Why would I?"

—Caroline Beckman, 20, adventurist and head of special projects for Suja

headfirst into the cookie jar (we've all been there!). Not only that, but when the body needs fuel and it doesn't get it, your blood sugar drops and your metabolism slows down. Translation: You stop burning calories, and the next time you do eat, your body is likely to store those calories as fat in anticipation of the next missed meal.

To avoid this, stay ahead of your hunger. Keep healthy snacks on hand (in your purse, car, gym bag, or office drawer) so you have nutritious in-crowd foods available when hunger strikes. Snack on protein and fiber between meals to keep your concentration sharp, your metabolism stoked, and your body burning usable energy.

Mix-and-Match Juices

All juices in the program are designed to be mix-and-match *within mealtimes*. This means that all of the reset and reinforce morning, midday, and early-evening juices are available to you, so long as you drink them within the appropriate mealtimes. We've designed the program this way because we understand that you'll likely develop a special taste for a select few, and we want you to feel free to drink as much as you want of the juices you enjoy the most!

This week's recipes are focused on restorative juices and foods that continue the process of removing waste and weight without taxing your digestion, while giving you a boost in energy to fuel a higher activity level and stimulate your brain. The recipes this week build upon last week. This makes shopping and food prep easy, and with the addition of savory nut butters and starchy sweet potatoes, for example, your meals will taste like totally new creations. If you're someone who likes to play the executive chef in your house, feel free to craft your own meals instead from the list of ingredients on this week's shopping list.

WEEK 2 MEAL PLAN

Each day this week, you will follow the same juice + meal plan for morning, midday, and early evening.

Morning

Start your day on an empty stomach, and rehydrate with a morning citrus juice (see the reinforce program juice recipes in chapter 13).

MORNING JUICE

Beet You to the Top, page 146

Balance, page 146

Thirty minutes later, or when hunger appears, you will eat your morning meal (see chapter 13). You're invited to prepare any of the suggested morning meals. This week, we've created three new morning meal recipes for you to choose from. You can eat them in whatever order you wish. If you want more options, you're invited to create your own morning meal instead by combining 4 ounces lean protein, unlimited fresh green veggies, and 1 medium fresh fruit *or* ½ cup starchy veggies and 1 tablespoon healthy fats from the week 2 shopping list. For vegetarians, combine ¾ cup legumes and ½ cup starchy veggies *or* 1 medium fresh fruit, unlimited fresh green veggies, and 1 tablespoon healthy oil *or* 2 tablespoons nuts *or* ⅓ avocado.

MORNING MEAL

Apple Pie That You Can't Buy, page 147

Sweet Potato Perfection, page 147

Surfer's Delight, page 148

If hunger appears between your morning and midday meals, see *Grab 'n' Go Snack Ideas* in chapter 13.

Custom Blends

If you're short on time in the kitchen, order a custom blend to go at your local juice bar or juice truck. We've simplified all of the juice recipes in the program to Juice Bar Blends so you can grab 'n' go. For blender users, we've made each recipe blender-friendly by adding a few key ingredients that will turn it into a smoothie (see chapter 13).

Midday

When you feel the need for something at midday, choose either of the juices below for a sweet dose of colorful plant nutrition. Both midday juices provide root-veggie fiber and antioxidants, and work to flush unusable waste through the liver.

Double the recipe (24 to 32 ounces) to generate enough hearty garden goodness for both your afternoon and evening juice hydration. Store your juice in an airtight container in the fridge, and be sure to fill it all the way to the top to prevent oxidation and nutrient loss.

MIDDAY JUICE

Crimson Berry, page 148

Life Line, page 149

Wait until you feel hungry again before you eat your midday meal (see chapter 13). Prepare a meal from the 3 recipes provided, or create your own midday meal by combining 4 ounces lean protein, unlimited fresh green veggies, and 1 medium fresh fruit *or* ½ cup starchy veggies and 1 tablespoon healthy fats from the week 2 shopping list. For vegetarians, combine ¾ cup legumes and ½ cup starchy veggies *or* 1 medium fresh fruit, unlimited fresh green veggies, and 1 table-spoon healthy oil *or* 2 tablespoons nuts *or* ⅓ avocado. If, in between your midday and early-evening meals, you feel the need for something more, choose one of the whole-food snack options (see *Grab 'n' Go Snack Ideas* in chapter 13).

Is This You?
I'm Too Short on Time to Cook!

"Everyone is short on time, myself included. I work long hours and when I'm not working I spend most of my time being physically active: surfing, skiing, or diving...rarely taking time to sit down and fuel up with a solid meal. I started juicing—making fresh-pressed juice as a daily meal supplement, to give my body needed nutrients without being weighed down, while at the same time keeping hydrated.

"I love making juice, often returning to my same simple recipes, such as apple, pineapple, collard greens, ginger and a little spearmint added for character. Integrating juice into my lifestyle has realigned my palate toward fresher, healthier foods and I've realized that the more I get away from not-so-healthy foods, the easier it is to avoid them. As a result, I don't crave stimulants like coffee, sugar, and alcohol as much. I sleep better and wake up more alert and ready for whatever happens in my day. I tell my friends, 'Just try it for a few days and see how you feel. Do you feel better? Then keep going.'"

—Todd Nicholson, 48, avid surfer, free diver, fisherman, and skier

MIDDAY MEAL

Roasted Ruby Salad, page 149

San Diego Sando, page 150

Hot Bod Hummus Plate, page 151

Early Evening

When you start to feel hungry again in late afternoon or early evening, drink the remaining 12 to 16 ounces of the green juice you prepared at midday.

EARLY-EVENING JUICE

Crimson Berry, page 148

Life Line, page 149

Thirty minutes later, or when hunger re-appears, prepare your evening meal (see chapter 13). Prepare a meal from the three recipes provided, or create your own meal by combining 4 ounces lean protein, unlimited fresh green veggies, and 1 medium fresh fruit *or* ½ cup starchy veggies and 1 tablespoon healthy fats from the week 2 shopping list. For vegetarians, combine ¾ cup legumes and ½ cup starchy veggies *or* 1 medium fresh fruit, unlimited fresh green veggies, and 1 tablespoon healthy oil *or* 2 tablespoons nuts

or ⅓ avocado. Consume this final whole-food meal of the day a minimum of two to three hours before bed to allow your body to fully digest *before* sleep.

EARLY-EVENING MEAL

Heavenly Halibut and Garlicky Greens, page 152

Liquid Sunshine, page 153

Kale-ifornia Salad 2.0, page 152

EAT MORE OF THESE IN-CROWD FOODS

This week, you will notice that many of the foods that were on last week's out-crowd list reappear on this week's in-crowd list. Note this week's yummy additions, listed in boldface:

Leafy greens: Arugula, baby greens, beet greens, collard greens, endive, fennel, kale, leeks, all lettuce (except iceberg), mustard greens, spinach, and Swiss chard

Vegetables: Artichokes, asparagus, bell peppers, broccoli, Brussels sprouts, cabbage (green and red), cauliflower, celery, cucumber, eggplant, jicama, mushrooms, onions, shallots, zucchini squash (green and yellow)—**plus beets, carrots, green garden peas, sugar snap peas, sweet potatoes, winter squash, yams**

Legumes: Lentils—**plus all beans, including black beans, butter beans, cannellini beans, chickpeas, great northern beans, kidney beans, lima beans, navy beans, pinto beans, white beans (note: refried beans are still off the list)**

Non-dairy Milk: Unsweetened almond milk, unsweetened coconut milk

Whole fruit: Avocado, grapefruit, lemon, lime, tomato—**plus low-glycemic whole fruits like berries (blackberries, blueberries, raspberries, strawberries), Granny Smith green apples, kiwi, nectarines, peaches, pears, pineapple (fresh in juices only), plums**

Lean proteins: Fish and shellfish (preferably wild-caught), canned fish like salmon, sardines, and tuna (no salt or oil added), organic turkey, organic chicken (skinless white meat), organic free-range whole eggs

Lunch meat: Nitrate-free, low-sodium, organic turkey, chicken

Good fats: Avocado oil, coconut oil, cold-pressed flax oil, extra-virgin olive oil, ghee (clarified butter)—**plus macadamia nut oil, walnut oil**

Unroasted seeds, nuts, and (sugar-free) nut butters: Almonds, macadamias, and walnuts; chia seeds and flaxseeds—**plus pine nuts, pumpkin seeds, sesame seeds, sunflower seeds, tahini**

Caffeine: Decaf coffee

Condiments: Apple cider vinegar, balsamic vinegar, white vinegar, Dijon mustard, non-GMO tamari (gluten-free soy sauce)

Herbs and spices: All

Sweeteners: Coconut water (unsweetened), stevia (organic or "whole leaf")

Live Colorfully

This week, you're adding a variety of colorful foods back to your plate.

ROOT VEGGIES

You crowded out root veggies for a solid week to help break your body's addiction to complex carbohydrates that can often convert to sugar, but they're the first foods to add back onto your plate because they're so rich in fiber, valuable vitamins, and antioxidants. In particular, carrots, butternut squash, and sweet potatoes have extremely high amounts of vitamin A, and beets are an amazing diuretic that will help your body continue to eliminate waste and stay regular.

When balanced with lean proteins and healthy fats, root veggies are a perfectly flavorful and filling addition to juices and whole-food meals. They provide the body with comforting complex carbs that fuel a higher activity level and act as wonderful brain food. This week, enjoy sweet roasted beets over salad, warm baked sweet potatoes with herbs and coconut oil or almond butter and cinnamon, and butternut squash as a delicious side to white fish or crumbled on a kale salad for a burst of sweetness. While they're higher in calories than green leafy veggies, these root vegetables are much lighter and easier to digest than grains, which is why they make

their comeback this second week as your main carbohydrate source.

LEGUMES

Legumes (with the exception of peanuts) are also back. As you gradually increase your intake of starch over the next 7 days, this fabulous source of plant protein and fiber makes the in-crowd list. Their unique combination of protein and carbohydrate can sometimes be hard for your body to handle, and yet they're masterful at boosting the body's energy and keeping blood sugar levels steady. As your body continues to adjust to a healthier equilibrium, beans will help you find the right balance.

WHOLE FRUIT

As far as we're concerned, fresh fruits are nature's perfect food. Their naturally occurring sugar, fructose and glucose, is easily digested by the body and made readily available for energy and fuel. Plus, fresh fruit makes life taste better! You limited your fruit intake to citrus in juices only during the first 7 days of the program, to help curb your sugar cravings and reset your taste buds for natural sweetness. But this week you can welcome back low-glycemic whole fruits like Granny

Smith green apples, peaches, pears, plums, and berries, which are all high in vitamins, minerals, phytochemicals, antioxidants, and fiber.

MORE HEALTHY FATS

This week, up your oil intake. We love whole macadamia nuts for their favorable ratio of omega-3 to omega-6 fatty acids, and walnuts for their vitamin E, iron, and calcium content—and the oils of both nuts are just as nutritious. They make a fabulous substitute for olive oil on salads and roasted veggies, infusing a deep nutty flavor along with offering a nutritional boost. Rich macadamia oil is very high in monounsaturated fats (higher than olive oil), and walnut oil has been shown to benefit cholesterol and reduce triglyceride levels. These oils have ellagic acid, which is an antioxidant that helps counter the effects of free radicals. Just like their whole-nut versions, these fats are very delicate and are easily damaged by heat, so make sure to use macadamia and walnut oil only on raw foods, on salads, or as a finishing oil on already cooked veggies.

Still craving grains this week? While you continue to take a break from grains and allow your digestive system to further rest and restore, add seeds and nut butters to foods this week to help satisfy your yearnings for heartier foods. Slather roasted sweet potato slices with almond butter. Miss that scoop of nutty quinoa on your salad? Add pumpkin and sunflower seeds to your greens instead for an extra craving-crushing protein boost and flavor depth. Choose organic, unroasted, unsweetened nut butters. Most commercial nut butters contain hydrogenated oils, sugar, corn syrup, and loads of salt, so read the ingredient list before heading to checkout. "All Natural" labels can be very misleading which is why we advocate making your own nut butters. This can save you a lot of money while also letting you experiment with flavor while knowing exactly what's in the jar.

COFFEE

Finally, coffee. *Ahhhh*, such a complex relationship! Most of us love coffee for the smell, the ritual, the deep-roasted flavor, and the antioxidants. But what's not to love are the jitters, the anxiousness, and the extra calories packed into many of the popular blended coffee drinks. So this week we'll meet you in the middle—organic decaf coffee. If you so desire, you can reintroduce your morning ritual without many of the undesirable side effects. Instead of sugar, sweeten it up with stevia; if you're someone who likes to add cream to your coffee, try adding a non-dairy, whole-food alternative like unsweetened, vitamin-rich almond milk or thick and creamy unsweetened coconut milk to your morning cup of Joe.

EAT LESS OF THESE OUT-CROWD FOODS

This week your focus is on reinforcing your new habits and keeping a healthy momentum going, so for the next 7 days we strongly suggest that you continue to crowd out the following foods, all of which tend to slow down your digestion and metabolism:

Grains: All, including gluten-free

Peanuts

Dried fruits

High-glycemic whole fruits: Apples (except Granny Smith), bananas, cantaloupe, cherries, dates, figs, grapes, honeydew melon, mangoes, oranges, papaya, pineapple (except in specified juices), tangerines, watermelon

High-starch veggies: Corn, white potatoes

Red meat: Bacon, beef, bison, duck, lamb, game meats, pork, rabbit, sausage (all)

Dairy: All

Refined and added sugars: Agave, all artificial sweeteners, beet sugar, brown rice syrup, brown sugar, coconut sugar, corn syrup, date sugar, evaporated cane juice, honey, jellies and jams, lactose, maple syrup, molasses, "raw" sugar, refined white sugar, Sucanat, turbinado sugar (stevia is the exception)

Bad fats: Canola oil, corn oil, cottonseed oil, grapeseed oil, hydrogenated or partially hydrogenated oil, margarine, peanut oil, safflower oil, soybean oil, sunflower oil

Soy products: Edamame, soybean oil, soy cheese, soy meats, soy milk, soy protein powder, soy yogurt, Tempeh, tofu

Alcohol

Processed and packaged foods

WELLNESS CHECK: RUNNING LOW? FILL UP ON OIL!

If at any point during week 2 you feel deprived, go heavier on natural oils. They will help add substance and complexity to the foods you're eating; in addition, when you add natural fats to your meals, you'll likely discover that you feel more full and satisfied. Natural oils are great for squashing a sugar craving, too, and by filling up on oil you may feel less hungry in between meals and feel the need to snack less. At 9 calories per gram versus 4 calories per gram for proteins and carbohydrates, they are a super source of energy; a little goes a long way. Start with adding an extra teaspoon or two to your salad or baked veggies and see how it makes you feel. That may be all you need.

WEEK 2 MOVE YOUR BODY: MODERATE EXERCISE

This week, kick up your level of physical activity. You're incorporating more complex carbs and proteins into your daily menus, and these fuel a higher activity level. Engage in brisk walking and light jogging; intermediate-level yoga and pilates requiring your strength, flexibility, and balance; or biking or swimming for a minimum of 30 to 60 minutes a day. These activities are a great complement to week 2 because they elevate your heart rate, blood circulation, and oxygen flow without taking the body's primary attention away from releasing waste, water retention, and repairing your digestion. If you can, get your exercise first thing in the morning. This elevates your heart rate for the rest of the day so you burn more calories at rest. Throughout the day, nourish and hydrate your body so it has fuel to burn and can work at its peak physical performance.

WEEK 2 SHOPPING LIST

Your shopping list this week looks just like last week's, with the exception of a handful of new delicious and satisfying additions like sweet potatoes and beets; peaches, plums and berries; lentils and sunflower seeds. You can create all the high-energy juices and whole-food recipes for weeks 1 and 2 from this all-inclusive list of ingredients. Notice that this week's additions are in bold to make grocery shopping a snap. As you continue to build upon this relatively simple list of fresh foods, you will quickly learn how to identify the most nutrient-dense fruits and vegetables, lean proteins, healthy fats, and complex carbohydrates to toss into your cart—and from there, how to make a variety of healthy dishes from them. Clean, lean, and colorful nutrition is relatively simple.

This Could Totally Be You:
Losing Those Last Stubborn Pounds

"I was a vegetarian when I became pregnant and then all of a sudden, I wanted nothing to do with veggies. All I wanted to eat was bagels and scrambled eggs— at every meal. Fast-forward nine months later and I had a 9 pound 4 ounce healthy baby boy—and also some extra weight to lose. That's when I discovered that by incorporating a couple of green juices into my post-pregnancy diet, along with a regular Spin class, I could easily drop the weight, and keep it off (don't hate me!). Juice gives me good energy, helps my metabolism and digestion, and has basically made me feel and look healthy again."

—Jessica Pratt, 29, wife, mother, and VP of natural sales–west, Suja

Fresh Produce

- Artichokes
- Arugula
- Asparagus
- Baby greens
- Bean sprouts
- Beets, beet greens
- Bell pepper
- Bok choy
- Broccoli
- Brussels sprouts
- Butter lettuce
- Cabbage (green and red)
- **Carrots**
- Cauliflower
- Celery
- Collard greens
- Cucumber
- Dandelion greens
- Eggplant
- Endive
- Fennel
- Green beans
- **Green garden peas**

- Green leaf lettuce
- Green onion
- Jicama
- Kale (Jacinto)
- Leeks
- Mushrooms (all)
- Pea sprouts
- Red bell pepper
- Red onion
- Romaine leaf lettuce
- Shallots
- Spinach
- **Sugar snap peas**
- **Sweet potato**
- Swiss chard
- Watercress
- **Winter squash (acorn, butternut, delicata, Hubbard, kabocha, pumpkin, spaghetti)**
- **Yams**
- Zucchini (green and yellow)

Week 2 Shopping Tip: Eat What You Love

Now that you're two weeks into the Suja Juice Solution, you've probably found some foods you love more than others. Were there any foods this week that never made it to your plate more than once because you didn't enjoy them as much as the foods you ran out of? Maybe you love asparagus and spinach but don't really enjoy broccoli. That's okay. In fact, we encourage you to stock your pantry and fridge with only the healthy foods that you *want* to eat again and again. Otherwise, if you have a particularly challenging day and all you have left in the fridge is Swiss chard, you may well end up ordering greasy takeout because you want to fill yourself up on something that quickly satisfies (even if it leaves your tummy not-so-satisfied an hour later). While variety has its merits, a simple menu may be the better course, especially when you're introducing healthy new habits. Purchase the foods and ingredients you know you'll actually prepare meals from, and build upon these foods and recipes week-to-week.

Fresh Whole Fruit

Apples (Granny Smith only)

Avocados

Berries (blackberry, blueberry, raspberry, strawberry)

Grapefruit

Kiwi

Lemons

Limes

Nectarines

Peaches

Pears

Pineapple (fresh in juices only)

Plums

Tomatoes (any)

Proteins

Beans (all except refried)— black beans, butter beans, cannellini beans, chickpeas, great northern beans, kidney beans, lentils, lima beans, navy beans, pinto beans, white beans

Canned salmon, sardines, and tuna (no oil or sodium)

Chicken (organic, skinless, white meat)

Eggs (organic, free-range)

Lunch meat: turkey and chicken (organic, low sodium, nitrate-free)

Turkey (organic, oven-roasted)

Wild-caught fish, shellfish (see page 31 for a list of the healthiest and safest choices)

Healthy Fats: Nuts, Seeds, and Butters

(Preferably unroasted, unsalted, and unsweetened)

Almonds and **almond butter**

Chia seeds

Flaxseeds

Macadamia nuts and **macadamia butter**

Pine nuts

Pumpkin seeds

Sesame seeds

Sunflower seeds and sunflower butter

Tahini

Walnuts

Fresh and Dried Herbs

Any and all! This week prepare juices and whole-food meals with your favorite dried or fresh herbs

Spices and Seasonings

Any and all! This week prepare juices and whole-food meals with your favorite dried or fresh spices and seasonings

Non-Dairy Milk

Almond milk (unsweetened)

Coconut milk (unsweetened)

Natural Sweeteners

Coconut water (unsweetened)

Shredded coconut (unsweetened)

Stevia (organic or "whole leaf")

Essential Oils and Pantry Staples

Apple cider vinegar

Avocado oil

Balsamic vinegar

Broth, vegetable and chicken (low sodium, no yeast or sugar)

Coconut oil

Cold-pressed flax oil

Decaffeinated coffee

Decaffeinated herbal tea

Dijon mustard

Extra-virgin olive oil

Ghee (clarified butter)

Macadamia nut oil

Tamari

Walnut oil

Vinegar

This week expect to feel cleaner, lighter, and even more balanced. The dense chlorophyll content of the leafy greens in the juices and meals you're preparing is oxygenating your blood and waking you up. Good-bye, hazy brain fog! Who knew simple foods with subtle flavors could be so rejuvenating and powerful?

You made it through two full weeks (14 days) of the Suja Juice Solution. Go, you! How do you feel? Super sharp, more focused and alert? Full of energy and a renewed zest for what your life has to offer? How's your appetite—did you wake up this morning craving nutrient-dense juice packed with vital amino acids, omegas, and antioxidants? Has your hunger for out-crowd foods like added sugars, saturated fats, and processed foods diminished to an even greater degree? Are you finding, instead, new satisfaction from simple clean foods that have a beautiful way of balancing and fueling your body and mind all day long? If your answer is *yes* (and we're hoping it is!), then you're going to love the next 7 days. Go, go, go!

HOW DO I DO THIS?

This week, you will recharge your body and mind for another 7 days of powerful transformation. You'll do this by adding more foods back onto your plate that fill you up with abundant physical and mental energy, renewed strength, and the motivation to continue forward toward optimal health. This week you will shift your focus from

CHAPTER 9

WEEK 3: 7 DAYS to RECHARGE

1 week, 2 steps, 3 juices

elimination and removal to replenishment and restoration. Welcome back gluten-free grains, dairy, and even desserts to your daily menu. Sweet! As you've been doing all along, for the next 7 days you will follow these simple steps:

Step 1. Add three juices every day.

Step 2. Crowd out not-so-healthy foods.

Over the course of the next 7 days, you will notice that the number of foods on your in-crowd list rounds up. You will gradually reintroduce foods that were crowded out in weeks 1 and 2, one at a time, to give your body a chance to readjust. To make this transition gentle and easy on your body, you're encouraged to try several "stepping-stone foods," like quinoa, goat's milk, and grass-fed beef. We call them stepping-stone foods because they substitute for their less-than-healthy rivals—wheat, rye, and barley; cow's-milk dairy; and industrial meat injected with hormones, chemicals, and antibiotics—foods that we hope you'll eventually step away from entirely. That being said, understand that every healthy

This Could Totally Be You:
Easily Managing Your Weight

"Four years ago I hit menopause. Sure enough, the weight gain wasn't far behind. In the past, I didn't have to do too much extra exercising or dieting to maintain my weight, but that was no longer the case. So I finally gave up my addiction to overprocessed foods and 'diet' drinks, and started drinking fresh juices instead. That's when the scale started to tip back in the right direction. I continue to enjoy juices throughout the week to help me get all the great nutrients I need to feel and look my best."

—Rebecca Vigil, 54, happy, healthy wife and mother

decision you make is a step forward. Try to make as many good steps forward as you can, knowing that regardless of what might slip past your lips (hey, we all cheat from time to time!), you're doing the best you can with what you've got, and that the high-powered, nutrient-dense juices you're drinking daily in addition to the fresh, whole foods you're consuming are doing absolute wonders for your body.

WEEK 3 MEAL PLAN

Each day this week, you will follow the same juice + meal plan for morning, midday, and early evening.

Morning

Choose from a fresh variety of fruit and vegetable juices along with a hearty new complement of whole-food meals that build upon last week's, making the next 7 days even more satisfying.

This week's juices and foods work together to recharge your body by providing more substantial building blocks like complex carbohydrates and a wider variety of proteins that help replenish your amino acid and energy stores in a healthful way after 14 days of flushing out your system.

You will start your day on an empty stomach, and rehydrate with a morning citrus juice.

Your Week 3: Recharge Meal Plan at a Glance

MORNING JUICE
Arise *or* Melon Spice

MORNING MEAL
Peaches and Cream *or* Sunrise Apple Pie *or* Awaken to Bacon

MIDDAY JUICE
Wholesome Harvest *or* Grounded

MIDDAY MEAL
Turned-Up Tabbouleh *or* Berry Nutty Salad *or* No-Flaw Slaw

EARLY-EVENING JUICE
Wholesome Harvest *or* Grounded

EARLY-EVENING MEAL
Amazin' Asian Sea Bass *or* Mexicali Mixer *or* Tangy 'n' Tropical Black Beans

DESSERT
Coconutty Lemon Burst Truffles *or* Brownies Done Better

MORNING JUICE

Arise, page 158

Melon Spice, page 158

Both of these morning elixirs are fantastic to consume on an empty stomach because they're efficient at neutralizing your body's acidity and flushing out the system. They also contain enzymes that aid in healthy digestion. And if that doesn't whet your appetite, these bright morning quenchers are an excellent source of vitamin C and manganese, which helps your body utilize nutrients and metabolize fats and carbohydrates for energy. It also helps the body regulate blood sugar.

Thirty minutes later, or when hunger appears, you will eat your morning meal.

You're invited to prepare any of the suggested morning meals, in whichever order you choose (see chapter 14), or create your own instead by combining 5 ounces animal protein from the in-crowd options, unlimited green veggies, ½ cup starchy veggies, legumes, or gluten-free grain and 1 tablespoon healthy oil *or* 2 tablespoons nuts *or* ⅓ avocado. For vegetarians, create your own morning meal by combining unlimited green veggies, ¾ cup legumes, and ½ cup starchy veggies *or* ½ cup gluten-free grains and 1 tablespoon healthy oil *or* 2 tablespoons nuts *or* ⅓ avocado.

MORNING MEAL

Peaches and Cream, page 159

Sunrise Apple Pie, page 159

Awaken to Bacon, page 160

Midday

When your belly starts making noise at midday, prepare either of the high-powered juices below. Double the recipe (24 ounces) to generate enough hearty, root-veggie goodness for both your afternoon and evening juice hydration. Store your juice in an airtight container in the fridge, and be sure to fill it all the way to the top to prevent oxidation and nutrient loss.

MIDDAY JUICE

Wholesome Harvest, page 160

Grounded, page 161

If hunger appears between your morning and midday meals, see *Grab 'n' Go Snack Ideas* in chapter 14.

Wait until you feel hungry again before you eat your midday meal. Choose from the three recipes provided, or create your own instead by combining 5 ounces animal protein from the in-crowd options, unlimited green veggies, and ½ cup starchy veggies, legumes, or gluten-free grains and 1 tablespoon healthy oil *or* 2 tablespoons nuts *or*

This Could Totally Be You:
Endless Health Benefits

"I have seen the health benefits of juicing personally. The benefits include increased energy, improved mental clarity, improved skin and hair condition, and general nutritional health.

"My children love the taste of fruit and vegetables, too. I cannot pour a juice without my children asking, 'Can I have some?'"

—Cambra Finch, PhD, 40, mother and clinical psychologist

⅓ avocado. For vegetarians, create your own meal by combining unlimited green veggies, ¾ cup legumes, and ½ cup starchy veggies *or* ½ cup gluten-free grains *or* 1 medium fresh fruit and 1 tablespoon healthy oil *or* 2 tablespoons nuts *or* ⅓ avocado. If you feel hungry in between your midday and early-evening meals, choose one of the grab 'n' go snack options.

MIDDAY MEAL

Turned-Up Tabbouleh, page 161

Berry Nutty Salad, page 162

No-Flaw Slaw, page 162

Early Evening

When you start to feel hungry again in late afternoon or early evening, drink the remaining 12 ounces of the green juice you prepared at midday.

EARLY-EVENING JUICE

Wholesome Harvest, page 160

Grounded, page 161

Thirty minutes later, or when hunger reappears, prepare your evening meal. Choose from the recipes provided, or create your own meal instead by combining 5 ounces animal protein from the in-crowd options, unlimited green veggies, and ½ cup starchy veggies, legumes, or gluten-free grains *or* 1 medium fresh fruit and 1 tablespoon healthy oil *or* 2 tablespoons nuts *or* ⅓ avocado. For vegetarians, create your own meal by combining unlimited green veggies, ¾ cup legumes, and ½ cup starchy veggies *or* ½ cup gluten-free grains *or* 1 medium fresh fruit and 1 tablespoon healthy oil *or* 2 tablespoons nuts *or* ⅓ avocado.

EARLY-EVENING MEAL

Amazin' Asian Sea Bass, page 163

Mexicali Mixer, page 164

Tangy 'n' Tropical Black Beans, page 164

Still hungry for more? Indulge in one of these good-for-you desserts—a great way to wind down at the end of your day.

DESSERT

Coconutty Lemon Burst Truffles, page 165

Brownies Done Better, page 165

Consume your final whole-food meal and optional dessert of the day a minimum of two to three hours before bed to allow your body to fully digest *before* sleep.

EAT MORE OF THESE IN-CROWD FOODS

For the next 7 days, fill up on the following in-crowd foods. Note this week's colorful and filling additions, listed in boldface:

Leafy greens: Arugula, baby greens, beet greens, collard greens, endive, fennel, kale, leeks, all lettuce (except iceberg), mustard greens, spinach, Swiss chard

Vegetables: Artichokes, asparagus, bean sprouts, beets, bell peppers, broccoli, Brussels sprouts, cabbage, carrots, cauliflower, celery, cucumber, eggplant, green garden peas, green beans, jicama, mushrooms, onions, shallots, snap peas, sweet potatoes, winter squash (acorn, butternut, delicata, Hubbard, kabocha, pumpkin, spaghetti), zucchini squash (green and yellow), yams

Legumes: All beans—**plus organic edamame (whole soybeans)**

Gluten free grains: Amaranth, brown rice, buckwheat, hemp seed, millet, quinoa, whole or steel-cut oats (Note: flours, packaged gluten-free crackers and bread, and whole wheat are still off the list!)

Non-dairy milks: Unsweetened almond milk, unsweetened coconut milk—**plus hazelnut milk**

Whole fruit: Avocado, berries (blackberries, blueberries, raspberries, strawberries), grapefruit, kiwi, lemon, lime, nectarines, peaches, pears, plums, and tomato—**plus all apples, bananas, cherries, figs, mangoes, oranges, papayas, and pineapple**

Lean proteins: Organic chicken and turkey (skinless white meat), organic free-range eggs, fish, and shellfish (preferably wild-caught or sustainably farmed), canned fish like salmon, sardines, or tuna (no salt or oil added)—**plus grass-fed bison, beef, and lamb; chicken and turkey sausages; nitrate-free turkey bacon**

Lunch meat: Nitrate-free, low-sodium, organic turkey, chicken

Dairy: Goat's butter; goat's and sheep's milk; unsweetened goat's and sheep's yogurt and kefir; goat's- and sheep's-milk cheeses

Good fats: Avocado oil, coconut oil, cold-pressed flax oil, extra-virgin olive oil, ghee (clarified butter), macadamia nut oil, walnut oil

Unroasted seeds, nuts, and (sugar-free) nut butters: Almonds, macadamias, pine nuts, and walnuts; chia seeds and flax-seeds; pumpkin seeds, sesame seeds, sunflower seeds; tahini—**plus Brazil nuts, hazelnuts, pecans**

Caffeine: Regular and decaf coffee

Condiments: Apple cider vinegar, balsamic vinegar, Dijon mustard, non-GMO tamari (gluten-free soy sauce), vinegar

Herbs and spices: All

Natural sweeteners: coconut water, stevia—**plus coconut palm sugar, date sugar, honey, maple syrup**

Epic Taste

This week, you're adding back to your plate a satisfying range of flavors to be sure to tickle your taste buds.

GRAINS

While grains are back, it's important to keep them gluten-free (for now) to ease your body back into digesting them. Enjoy gluten-free grains like protein- and iron-packed quinoa, B-vitamin-rich millet, robust and earthy buckwheat, omega-3 superstar hemp seed, and light pepper amaranth. Notice how you feel after consuming them. Unlike wheat, rye, and barley, which often irritate and slow digestion, these gluten-free grain options may sit just right with you. You may feel less tired after eating them, and your tummy may feel lighter and more comfortable after a meal. And while gluten-free grains are on this week's in-crowd list, we encourage you to crowd out processed gluten-free foods like crackers and bread. If this is a confusing distinction, we feel you. Each one of us has experienced frustration in our individual quests for diet and nutrition information. Meat or no meat, grains or no grains, fruit or no fruit . . . ahhh! What's a health-conscious person to do? In this case, processed gluten-free foods like crackers, pretzels, and most breads are still off the list because most have little to no fiber, which means they don't fill you up for long. In fact, they can actually leave you feeling hungry for more. They also lack the protein that helps keep your blood sugar levels and healthy metabolism in check. And many gluten-free products are high in calories and added sugar, which can lead to weight gain. All in all—processed gluten-free products don't help you look and feel your best, so swap 'em out for pure and simple gluten-free grains.

RED MEAT

Grass-fed beef and other more substantial proteins like bison and lamb will add abundance to your plate this week. Choose grass-fed meats over grain-fed meats for several reasons—they're much lower in fat than grain-fed meats and also much higher in healthy omega-3 fatty acids due to the animals' almost exclusive green diet. Grass-fed meat is also four times higher than grain-fed in vitamin E, which is believed to be a potent anti-aging antioxidant. Overall, grass-fed cows are typically much healthier than commercially raised, grain-fed cows that are fed

large amounts of corn and soy that are difficult for them to digest. The result is feedlot bloat, which is responsible for the death of thousands of cattle annually. What's more, commercially raised cows are often injected with hormones (up to 90 percent) to help them grow as large as possible, along with antibiotics to prevent sickness and disease.

DAIRY

If you've been missing your yogurt and cheese, this is the week you've been waiting for. While we encourage you to continue to leave cow's milk on the shelf, you can add the creaminess of sheep's and goat's cheese, milk, butter, and yogurt into your diet this week. These products can easily be found in any standard natural market; Whole Foods, for instance, regularly carries two or three brands of each variety. Both sheep's and goat's milk make the in-crowd list this week because their molecular structure is very similar to that of human mother's milk, which our bodies were designed to recognize and digest. Additionally, the fat globules in cow's milk are all different sizes, and this makes extra work for your body to break down, whereas the fat globules in goat's and sheep's milk are all the same size, allowing for more fluid breakdown, absorption, and assimilation. Finally, goats do not respond to the human growth hormone (rBGH), so their milk is generally cleaner than conventional cow's-milk products that are often rBGH-treated.

NUTS

Pecans, hazelnuts, and Brazil nuts are higher in omega-6 content than walnuts and macadamias and are more acidic than almonds, so you took a break from them for a solid two weeks. But now that you understand proper portion control for nuts, you can add these guys back into your snack mix; they're great sources of plant protein, vitamins, and minerals.

NATURAL SWEETENERS

Now that you've given your sweet tooth a 14-day rest and your sensitivity to sugar has been reset, you may welcome back a few of our favorite natural sweeteners. In moderation, you can enjoy coconut palm sugar, date sugar, honey, and maple syrup. These natural sweeteners rank low on the glycemic index— they don't make a mad dash into your bloodstream and spike your blood sugar levels at the rate processed sugars do. Rather, these satisfying natural sweeteners break down to easily digestible glucose, which helps keep your blood sugar levels stable. We love coconut palm sugar for its molasses-y flavor and nutritional profile. It contains potassium, magnesium, zinc, and iron and is a natural source of the B vitamins. Date sugar, which is nothing more than dried dates ground into a powder, ranks high in antioxidants. In fact, researchers from the National Institutes of Health have ranked it the top sweetener out of 12 in antioxidant content. Natural honey has its perks as well. Especially if bought locally, it's commonly used to improve allergies, boost immunity, and soothe scratchy throats. If you can find it, we recommend organic, raw honey. Unlike conventional honey that's ultra-filtered, raw honey still has all the pollen, vitamins, antioxidants, and enzymes intact. Pure maple syrup is also a delicious addition this week, with high amounts of antioxidants, zinc, and the trace mineral manganese. It also contains calcium, potassium, sodium, and copper and has the same beneficial classes of polyphenols found in dark-colored foods like berries, tea, red wine, and tomatoes.

CAFFEINE

If you're a coffee or tea drinker, you can make the switch this week from decaf back to regular if you choose. Allow yourself one piping cup a day first thing in the morning, *before your first juice*. Drinking your coffee or tea before your first juice is important because the juices are very hydrating and alkalizing, while coffee and black tea are very dehydrating and acidic. By drinking your coffee or tea first, before alkalizing and hydrating with juice, the juice is able to do its job better. Your body can reap all the benefits of the juice without the interference of dehydrating and acidic caffeine.

If you do reintroduce caffeine this week, take careful notice of how it makes you feel. You'll likely be much more aware of the jolt now that you've been without it for two weeks and be satisfied with just one cup. If you can keep it to one cup in the morning, that's a perfectly acceptable way to partake in your morning ritual and benefit from its antioxidants without the detriments of over-stimulation of the adrenals and heart from multiple caffeine jolts per day.

Did You Know Magnesium-Dense Foods Can Counteract the Caffeine Jitters?

If you return to caffeine this week and feel the effects of it coming back too strong (your heart starts a-thumping, for instance, and your palms start sweating), integrate magnesium-rich foods into your next snack or meal. Spinach, pumpkin seeds, lentils, avocados, bananas, and brown rice are all magnesium-rich, helping to relax the nervous system and loosen tight muscles.

EDAMAME

All soy products were in the out-crowd for the last two weeks to give your body the optimal conditions to release waste, rest, and reset, but now you can add non-GMO edamame back into your diet. Edamame is the whole soybean and the least processed form of soy. It's also less concentrated than soy isolates, so the estrogenic effects on the body are not as high. Whole soybeans contain manganese, selenium, copper, potassium, phosphorous, magnesium, iron, calcium, B vitamins, and vitamin K. They are also a great source of fiber. Consume them in moderation, but they're perfectly acceptable as a healthy snack or salad garnish.

EAT LESS OF THESE OUT-CROWD FOODS

In addition to processed gluten-free products, this week we suggest that you continue to crowd out the super-slow-down stuff like processed foods, dried fruit, and soy products, which tend to be addictive and irritating to most of us. By now—14 days into the program—you may have already gotten into an automatic habit of crowding out these not-so-good-for-you foods without even thinking about it. If so, that's awesome! If not, be mindful of crowding out the following list of foods over the next 7 days:

Grains: Wheat, rye, barley, spelt, kamut, and their flours

Peanuts

Dried fruits: All

High-glycemic whole fruits: Dates, cantaloupe, honeydew melon, grapes, watermelon

High-starch veggies: Corn, white potatoes

Red meat: Pork

Dairy: Cow's milk

Refined and non-fruit sugar: Agave, processed white sugar

Bad fats: Canola oil, corn oil, cottonseed oil, grapeseed oil, hydrogenated and partially hydrogenated oil, margarine, peanut oil, safflower oil, soybean oil, sunflower oil

Soy products: Soybean oil, soy cheese, soy meats, soy milk, soy protein powder, soy yogurt, Tempeh, tofu

Alcohol

Processed and packaged foods

WELLNESS CHECK: ENJOY RICHNESS IN MODERATION

This week, as you welcome back dairy, coffee, desserts, and red meat into your healthier lifestyle, your challenge will be to reintroduce them in moderation. While it may be tempting to load up on these heavier foods now that you've been given the go-ahead to eat them—take it easy. Remind yourself that you can enjoy a juicy steak, a deep-roasted cup of coffee, and a sweet treat at the end of a meal without going off the deep end. In fact, you'll soon discover that it's quite easy to savor these flavorful foods within the context of a balanced meal. This is exactly what you've been learning to do from the start of the program! The simple foods you ate during week 1 became the baseline from which all other meals were built. Once you reset and rebalanced your system, you slowly built up—maintaining that gentle balance while adding more complex foods back onto your plate. Perhaps without even realizing it, you now know how to eat in moderation,

in a way that maintains a healthy balance of lean protein, carbohydrate, healthy fats, and natural sweetness. If you're in any doubt that you're striking the right balance, ask yourself: *What can I add or subtract from this meal to make it more balanced and easy for my body to digest?* You may be surprised at how quickly you come up with an answer.

WEEK 3 MOVE YOUR BODY: MODERATE EXERCISE

This week, add some heat-inducing cardio back into your exercise routine. With all the nutrient-dense juice and complex foods you've been consuming this week, you should feel revitalized, reinvigorated, and full of energy to burn. Running, hiking, Bikram or other styles of heated yoga, and Zumba or cardio-pump classes including moderate strength training are all great complements to week 3. Your body can now support the higher level of exertion that will promote the formation of new muscles, stoke a healthy metabolism, and increase your cardiovascular capacity for better endurance. While it's by no means necessary, aim to get in a killer 60-minute workout at least three days this week, and remember that when you exercise first thing in the morning, you stoke your metabolism so that you're efficiently burning fuel throughout the day.

If you feel hungry after being physically active, *eat*! There is no need to deprive yourself by suffering through too great a calorie deficit.

This Could Totally Be You:
Juice Helps Keep My Lifestyle on Track

"*I consider myself a cyclist in a business person's body. Pedal power to body weight ratio is all-important to excelling in cycling. The problem is that late night entertaining, sitting on airplanes and in airports for hours on end, stress induced eating, etc. . . . are all endemic to the career I have chosen. If I did not need a job to pay for all my 'non-professional' cycling, life would be grand. However that is not the case and I need to work. That is why when I'm not traveling for work I drink juice regularly to reset my body.*

"*For me, this convinces my body that it does not need to binge diet in order to stay fit. I really do feel like it has helped train my stomach to know when it is full and to stop the cravings that cause so many weight gain issues. The result has been that over the last few years I have maintained a steady even-keel weight. And that has not been the case before I started drinking more juice to complement and sometimes supplement meals. The only thing that frustrates me is that many of my friends that struggle with slow creeping weight gain caused by 'life' have not adopted my same healthy practices!*"

—David Vigil, 54, hard-core cyclist and CEO of Antenna79

Incorporate a pre- or post-workout juice into your day (see the recipes in chapter 14) to hydrate on a deep cellular level and replenish your glycogen stores. Listen to your body and give it what it needs to stay balanced.

WEEK 3 SHOPPING LIST

This week your shopping list is a bit longer, with foods like dairy, grains, and red meats tacked on. Notice again that this week's additions are in bold to help make shopping quick and easy. You can now create all the high-energy juices and whole-food recipes for the past *three* weeks from this all-inclusive list of fresh foods and ingredients.

Fresh Produce

- Artichokes
- Arugula
- Asparagus
- Baby greens
- Bean sprouts
- Beets, beet greens
- Bell pepper
- Bok choy
- Broccoli
- Brussels sprouts
- Butter lettuce
- Cabbage (green and red)
- Carrots
- Cauliflower
- Celery
- Collard greens
- Cucumber
- Dandelion greens
- Eggplant
- Endive
- Fennel
- Green beans
- Green garden peas
- Green leaf lettuce
- Green onion
- Jicama
- Kale
- Leeks
- Mushrooms
- Pea sprouts
- Red onion
- Romaine leaf lettuce
- Shallots
- Spinach
- Sugar snap peas
- Sweet potato
- Swiss chard
- Watercress
- Winter squash (acorn, butternut, delicata, Hubbard, kabocha, pumpkin, spaghetti)
- Yams
- Zucchini (green and yellow)

Fresh Whole Fruit

- **Apples (all)**
- Avocados
- **Bananas**
- Berries (blackberry, blueberry, raspberry, strawberry)
- **Cherries**
- **Figs**
- Grapefruit
- Kiwi
- Lemons
- Limes
- **Mangoes**
- **Melon (in juices only)**
- Nectarines
- **Oranges**
- **Papaya**
- Peaches
- Pears
- **Pineapple**
- Plums
- Tomatoes (any)

Week 3 Shopping Tip: Bulk Bins

Now that you've gotten into a comfortable and juicy groove of loading up on fresh, organic produce at the farmer's market and hitting the grocery store each week with an organized list of healthy staples that you enjoy cooking with and eating, it's time to optimize your shopping strategy. Bulk bins will help you do this. They help you cut costs because you can purchase only the quantity you need at reduced bulk-bin prices. We recommend buying all of your nuts, grains, and seeds from the bulk bins. Buying in bulk also provides you with an excuse to try something new, like dark-chocolate-covered almonds rolled in coconut (to die for!), without buying and, um, eating, a whole container of them.

Proteins

Beans (all)— black beans, butter beans, cannellini beans, chickpeas, **edamame** soybeans, great northern beans, kidney beans, lentils, lima beans, navy beans, pinto beans, white beans

Beef (grass-fed)

Bison (grass-fed)

Canned salmon, sardines, or tuna (no oil or sodium)

Chicken (organic, skinless, white meat) and organic **chicken sausage**

Eggs (organic, free-range)

Lamb (grass-fed)

Lunch meat turkey and chicken (organic, low sodium, nitrate-free)

Turkey (organic, oven-roasted), organic **turkey sausage, and turkey bacon (nitrate-free)**

Wild-caught or sustainably farmed fish, shellfish (see page 31 for a list of the healthiest and safest choices)

Gluten-Free Grains

Amaranth

Brown rice

Buckwheat

Hemp seed

Millet

Oat bran

Quinoa

Whole or steel-cut oats

Dairy

Goat's milk, butter, cheese, yogurt and kefir (unsweetened)

Sheep's milk, butter, cheese, yogurt and kefir (unsweetened)

Healthy Fats: Nuts, Seeds, and Butters

(Preferably unroasted, unsalted, and unsweetened)

Almonds and almond butter

Brazil nuts

Chia seeds

Flaxseeds

Hazelnuts

Macadamia nuts and macadamia butter

Pecans

Pine nuts

Pumpkin seeds

Sesame seeds

Sunflower seeds and sunflower butter

Tahini

Walnuts

Fresh and Dried Herbs

Any and all! This week prepare juices and whole-food meals with your favorite dried or fresh herbs

Spices and Seasonings

Any and all! This week prepare juices and whole-food meals with your favorite dried or fresh spices and seasonings

Natural Sweeteners and non-dairy milks

Almond milk (unsweetened)

Cacao powder

Coconut milk (unsweetened)

Coconut palm sugar

Coconut water (unsweetened)

Date sugar

Hazelnut milk (unsweetened)

Honey (preferably raw)

Maple syrup

Shredded coconut (unsweetened)

Stevia (organic or "whole leaf")

Essential Oils and Pantry Staples

Apple cider vinegar

Avocado oil

Balsamic vinegar

Broth, vegetable and chicken (low sodium, no yeast or sugar)

Caffeinated coffee

Caffeinated herbal tea

Coconut oil

Cold-pressed flax oil

Dijon mustard

Extra-virgin olive oil

Ghee (clarified butter)

Macadamia nut oil

Miso

Tamari

Walnut oil

Vinegar

This week's combination of fresh juices and whole foods should recharge your physical and mental energy reserves while satisfying your hunger for heavier, more complex foods. As you fill up on this week's in-crowd foods, pause to check in with your body. Become mindful of what feels good and what doesn't, and understand that just because we've moved some heavier foods back onto your plate doesn't mean they have to stay there. In other words, if a food isn't serving you, do yourself a favor and pass.

Hey superstar, you completed 3 weeks of the Suja Juice Solution. You're up to 21 days of clean, lean living. How do you feel now? Replenished and recharged? Sweetly satisfied and fulfilled after loading some heavier protein, hearty grains, and tropical fruits back onto your plate? By slowly reintroducing these foods after a legit hiatus, you may have noticed flavors, textures, and sensitivities you hadn't before because you'd always eaten them as a matter of course. For example, after abstaining from creamy and rich dairy for two weeks, how did your body react to sheep's and goat's milk? Any bloating or upset tummy? It's not uncommon at this point of the program to recognize new sensitivities to foods you've traditionally eaten. With the reintroduction of grass-fed beef and other heavier proteins, you may have experienced a sense of sluggishness or fatigue. Or you may have felt a surge of physical energy. After adding just one cup of coffee back into your morning routine, you may have noticed a mental shift from calm and clear to a little more anxious, even stressed. Or a little caffeine jolt may have felt fantastic! Either way, it's important to notice how you feel as you continue to reintroduce

CHAPTER 10

WEEK 4: 7 DAYS to RENEW

1 week, 2 steps, 3 juices

more complex foods and substances back into your life. This information will be helpful to you this week, and moving forward into the future.

HOW DO I DO THIS?

The next 7 days should feel easy and breezy. This week, it's not required that you crowd out any foods; just make your preferred choices, meal by meal. That's right—eat as you would on a typical day, although don't be too surprised to discover that after 21 days of hydrating with nutrient-dense juices and eating whole-food nutrition, what was once typical for you has shifted. After three weeks of resetting, fortifying, and recharging your body and mind, you may have a *new* normal. This week, as you select foods, we encourage you to take the following simple step:

One step: Add three juices every day.

That's right, just one step! As you've been doing all along, continue to consume three delicious, organic juices—one before each of your three meals. You'll have additional juices to choose from this week, all packed with fruits, vegetables, amino acids, omegas, and antioxidants, providing you with a convenient way to drink a substantial amount of the daily nutrients your body needs to maintain overall, vibrant health. By continuing to drink

This Could Totally Be You:
Fewer Cravings, More Energy

"Gone are the unhealthy cravings that used to drag me down. It is so rewarding to not even want an unhealthy snack. I crave juice instead! It fills me up and it provides that added kick of energy so needed mid-morning and afternoon."

—Diane Hamilton, 55, cyclist and seasoned traveler

high-powered juice before each of your morning, midday, and early-evening meals, our bet is that *by your own choosing* you'll make healthier food choices without thinking much about it. Most all of us at Suja have experienced firsthand how this natural evolution works—by consuming more nutrient-dense vegetable and fruit juice before you sit down to eat, you automatically eat less of the out-crowd stuff because you're so full of clean nourishment and fuel. Take it from us—it's a pretty amazing feeling. This week, you may even find yourself turning away from foods you used to always love because you *crave* a healthier alternative instead.

WEEK 4 MEAL PLAN

Each day this week, you will follow the same juice + meal plan for morning, midday, and early evening.

Morning

Start your day on an empty stomach, and rehydrate with a morning citrus juice. In a hurry? No problem. This week, you don't need to fire up your juicer and make a complex blend every morning. Your body will benefit

---

Your Week 4: Renew Meal Plan at a Glance

MORNING JUICE

Mediterranean *or* Watermelon Breeze

MORNING MEAL

Banana Cream Chia Oatmeal *or* Sunny Side Sammy *or* Better Bacon Omelet

MIDDAY JUICE

The Greens *or* Island Greens

MIDDAY MEAL

Bliss Burgers *or* Mediterranean Medley *or* Never-Fail Kale Salad

EARLY-EVENING JUICE

The Greens *or* Island Greens

EARLY-EVENING MEAL

Beach Bum Burritacos *or* Seared Scallops in the Sand *or* Oh My Thai Bowl

DESSERT

Sunflower Power Cookies *or* Cacao Almond Super Snacks

---

from a simple alkalizing and digestion-stimulating citrus kick. Squeeze lemon in hot or cold water with a splash of apple cider vinegar and a dash of cayenne, a touch of ginger, or a pinch of turmeric. You're good to go!

MORNING JUICE

Mediterranean, page 170

Watermelon Breeze, page 170

Thirty minutes later, or when hunger appears, you will eat your morning meal. While you're invited to eat meals of your choosing this week, in an effort to help you maintain healthy portions and a balanced plate, we've gone ahead and created another week's worth of recipes to make meal preparation a no-brainer. Again, if these options don't tantalize your taste buds, then create your own meals instead. For meat eaters, we suggest combining 5 ounces animal protein from the in-crowd options, unlimited green veggies, and ¾ cup starchy veggies, *or* legumes, *or*

Custom Blends

No time to fire up the juicer? Order a juice from your local juice bar or juice truck. We've converted all of the juice recipes in the program to Juice Bar Blends so you can simply grab 'n' go. For blender users, we've made each recipe blender-friendly by adding a few key ingredients that will turn it into a smoothie (see chapter 15).

gluten-free grains, and 1 tablespoon healthy oil *or* 2 tablespoons nuts *or* ⅓ avocado. If you're a vegetarian, combine unlimited green veggies with one of the following: ¾ cup legumes, ¾ cup starchy veggies, ¾ cup gluten-free grains; 1 tablespoon healthy oil *or* 2 tablespoons nuts *or* ⅓ avocado.

MORNING MEAL

Banana Cream Chia Oatmeal, page 171

Sunny Side Sammy, page 171

Better Bacon Omelet, page 172

If hunger appears between your morning and midday meals, see *Grab 'n' Go Snack Ideas* in chapter 15.

Midday

When you feel the need for something at midday, prepare either of the high-powered green juices below. They're like green lightning to your system! These garden-fresh, all-purpose juices provide your body with a mega-dose of concentrated green nutrition that's easy for your body to quickly absorb. Consider them your liquid daily multivitamin. The oxygenating chlorophyll, phytochemicals, vitamins, minerals, amino acids, and antioxidants are everything you need to feel your best and energize your body, blood cells, and brain.

MIDDAY JUICE

The Greens, page 173

Island Greens, page 173

Double the recipe (16 ounces) to generate enough green goodness for both your afternoon and evening juice therapy. Store your juice in an airtight container in the fridge, and be sure to fill it all the way to the top to prevent oxidation and nutrient loss.

Thirty minutes later, or when hunger reappears, prepare your midday meal. Prepare any of the three recipes provided, or create your own by combining 5 ounces animal protein from the in-crowd options, unlimited green veggies, and ¾ cup starchy veggies *or* legumes *or* gluten-free grains *or* 1 tablespoon healthy oil *or* 2 tablespoons nuts *or* ⅓ avocado. If you're a vegetarian, combine unlimited green veggies and one of the following: ¾ cup legumes, ¾ cup starchy veggies, ¾ cup gluten-free grains; 1 tablespoon healthy oil *or* 2 tablespoons nuts *or* ⅓ avocado.

Mix-and-Match Juices

All juices in the program are designed to be mix-and-match *within mealtimes*. This means that all of the morning, midday, and early-evening juices throughout weeks 1-4 are available to you so long as you drink them within the appropriate mealtimes. We've designed the program this way because we understand that you'll likely develop a special taste for a select few, and we want you to feel free to drink as much as you want of the juices you enjoy the most!

MIDDAY MEAL

Bliss Burgers, page 174

Mediterranean Medley, page 175

Never-Fail Kale Salad, page 176

If, in between your midday and early-evening meal, you feel hungry, choose a whole-food snack.

EARLY EVENING

When you start to feel hungry again in late afternoon or early evening, drink the remaining 8 ounces of the green juice you prepared at midday. Thirty minutes later, or when hunger reappears, prepare your evening meal. Prepare any of the three recipes provided, or create your own meal by combining 5 ounces animal protein from the in-crowd options, unlimited green veggies, and ¾ cup starchy veggies *or* legumes *or* gluten-free grains *or* 1 tablespoon healthy oil *or* 2 tablespoons nuts *or* ⅓ avocado. If you're a vegetarian, combine unlimited green veggies and one of the following: ¾ cup legumes, ¾ cup starchy veggies, ¾ cup gluten-free grains; 1 tablespoon healthy oil *or* 2 tablespoons nuts *or* ⅓ avocado. Consume this final whole-foods meal and the optional dessert of the day a minimum of two to three hours before bed to allow your body to fully digest *before* sleep.

EARLY-EVENING MEAL

Beach Bum Burritacos, page 176

Seared Scallops in the Sand, page 177

Oh My Thai Bowl, page 178

Still hungry for more? Sip on a superfood milk shake (see chapter 16) or dive into one of the sin-free sweets below (see chapter 15).

DESSERT

Sunflower Power Cookies, page 179

Cacao Almond Super Snacks, page 180

FILL UP ON THESE IN-CROWD FOODS

Leafy greens: All

Vegetables: All

Legumes: All except peanuts

Grains: Amaranth, barley, brown rice, buckwheat, hemp seed, kamut, millet, quinoa, rye, spelt, wheat, whole or steel-cut oats

Non-dairy milks: Unsweetened coconut, almond, cashew, and hazelnut milk

Whole fruit: All

Proteins: Organic turkey and chicken (skinless white meat); organic free-range eggs, fish, and shellfish (preferably wild-caught); canned fish like salmon, sardines, and tuna (no salt or oil added); grass-fed beef, bison, lamb, **pork**; chicken, pork, and turkey sausage; **nitrate-free pork, beef, or turkey bacon; beef and turkey jerky (nitrate-free, unsweetened), organic duck, rabbit, and game meats**

Lunch meat: turkey, chicken, **ham** (organic, low sodium, nitrate-free)

Dairy: Cow's, goat's, and sheep's milk; unsweetened **cow's,** goat's, and sheep's yogurt; unsweetened **cow's,** goat's, and sheep's kefir; **cow's-,** goat's-, and sheep's-milk cheeses (all preferably organic and hormone-free), cow's-, goat's-, and sheep's-milk butter

Good fats: Avocado oil, coconut oil, flax oil, ghee (clarified butter), macadamia nut oil, olive oil, walnut oil

Unroasted seeds, nuts, and (sugar-free) nut butters: All

Caffeine: Coffee, tea

Alcohol

Condiments: Dijon mustard, non-GMO tamari (gluten-free soy sauce), and all vinegars

Herbs, spices, and natural sweeteners: All fresh and dried herbs and spices; coconut palm sugar, coconut water, date sugar, honey, maple syrup, **molasses,** stevia

CELE-BRATE!

As you can see, your in-crowd list has stretched even longer this week—it practically wraps around the block! Pork, rabbit, and heavier dark meats like duck are back on the menu. Cow's-milk dairy and all grains including wheat, rye, barley, spelt, and kamut are also once again available to you. So if you're someone who's always enjoyed a big bowl of O's with cow's milk in the morning, pour yourself one and dig in! Dates and cashews, both high in natural sugars and starch, are added back onto the list this week now that you've curbed your sweet tooth and learned portion control. Corn also makes a comeback.

This Could Totally Be You:
Choosing Wellness Whatever the Cost

"In college I played tennis, which meant traveling throughout the school term with my teammates. We'd often stop for meals, late at night and at fast-food restaurants or 24-hour diners with limited options. Most of my teammates didn't mind this—eating junk was fun—but I suffered from pretty serious gluten and dairy allergies so fun would quickly turn to pain. I knew that if I ate what the rest of my team ate, I'd be sick. I remember thinking, All my friends can eat whatever they want, and I have to travel with 'safe' foods like carrot sticks and nuts. Not much fun for me!

"I really felt like my choices were limited. The solution to my problem came when I discovered green juice in my early twenties. Juice did not upset my stomach and I swear, after drinking them my body started to crave them like I needed the vitamin rush. While I still have stomach issues—it's an ongoing struggle that I'll always have to be mindful of—my new diet of healthy foods and juicing has definitely helped. Some of my friends say, 'But juice is too expensive,' and I tell them that you can be healthy on a budget. You just have to choose how you want to spend your money. I'd rather splurge on organic food and juice than on fancy coffee drinks or cocktails out at a bar. My money goes towards my health."

—Bella Tumini, 24, travel enthusiast and brand manager, Suja

Organic, non-GMO corn on the cob, sprouted corn tortillas, and organic corn chips enjoyed in moderation are a perfectly acceptable addition at this point in the program. A handful of organic, non-GMO whole corn kernels in salads, tacos, and casseroles can bulk up your dishes without being detrimental to your blood sugar and body chemistry. And finally, you may indulge in a low-cal cocktail in the evening. To help get the party started, we've created and included an original selection of Suja Spirits in the full recipe section (see chapter 16). The Glowing Margagreena will light you up!

As you reintroduce these foods and substances back into your diet, remember to check in with how they make you feel. Think of this final week of the program as your beta test for the lifestyle you want to maintain for weeks, months, and years ahead. With this in mind, become hyperaware of what sits well in your body and what doesn't. If you notice that after you eat whole wheat, for example, your digestion feels sluggish, or if you feel bloated, gassy, or fatigued, consider backing off the all-gluten grains and substituting gluten-free quinoa or brown rice. Refer back to the list of "stepping-stone" foods from week 3 (chapter 9). They may better serve you. Continue to be ever mindful of what feels right in your body and eat more of those foods. Eventually, you will customize a nutritional plan that works best for your body and lifestyle—a way to eat day-to-day that is satisfying, healthy, and thereby easy to sustain once you've finished the program.

EAT LESS OF THESE OUT-CROWD FOODS

While it's not required that you crowd out anything this week, we do have a short list of foods you may want to continue to leave off your shopping list. These foods really do nothing more than pack a detrimental punch to your waistline and digestion. Not only that, but they also tend to be powerfully addictive. Consider removing them from your diet this week, and perhaps stepping away from them for the long term. The longer you go without eating them, the less of a hold they'll have on you. Eventually, you'll break your attachment to them completely.

Refined white sugar, agave, corn syrup and high-fructose corn syrup

Soy products: Soybean oil, soy cheese, soy meats, soy milk, soy protein powder, soy yogurt, Tempeh, tofu

Dried fruit

White flour

Peanuts, including peanut butter

Bad fats: Canola oil, corn oil, cottonseed oil, grapeseed oil, hydrogenated and partially hydrogenated oil, margarine, peanut oil, safflower oil, soybean oil, sunflower oil

Processed foods

That's it. You can totally live without these foods—at least for most of the time, right? Nothing is forever, so if you find yourself at a restaurant that uses canola oil—chill. No need to sweat it. Simply make a conscious decision to eat healthier at your next meal. What's so cool about having stuck with the program this far is that now, your body can handle an out-crowd moment because it's a much more efficient machine. You've given your digestive tract a significant break

to eliminate waste that may have been lining and clogging up its interior, and reduce the bad bacteria that feed on sugar. Healthy gut bacteria with a higher ratio of the good guys means better digestion, so one gunky meal isn't going to hang around the way it would have if you were still overloading your body with these kinds of meals on a daily basis. By eating well the majority of the time, you are nourishing the organs and cells with the nutrients they need to efficiently do their jobs, even when they get faced with a less-than-optimal meal every so often. What we mean to say is that moving forward, you can be flexible and enjoy more freedom in the variety of foods you choose to eat day-to-day.

WELLNESS CHECK: HOLD ON TO THAT AWESOME FEELING!

By the end of this week, we hope you feel like a brand spankin' shiny new version of yourself! You've likely lost excess weight, given your metabolism a nice kick in the rear,

Is This You?
I'll Always Love My Meat and Potatoes

"I'm from Texas. I'm a meat and potatoes kind of guy. I'm also a bodybuilder, and so keeping a healthy diet and exercising regularly is something I've always done. Still, I never juiced or cleansed or did any of that funky stuff. In fact, I've never much liked juice because most of it is from concentrate, high in sugar and low on natural fruit. But then I tasted organic, natural, cold-pressed juices. Wow. They gave me a huge boost, more than I ever got from caffeine or energy drinks. Now I drink at least two bottles a day. I still eat a high protein, low carb, and low fat diet. In fact, I haven't changed my diet that much at all except now I've added juice to the mix, and I feel better than I ever have."

—Kurt Cahill, 47, avid BBQ eater, [former] bodybuilder, and Suja COO

noticed clearer skin and brighter eyes, and gotten some much-needed sleep. You've probably also been smiling a lot more due to a healthy boost of energy and self-esteem. This awesome feeling is what you want to hold on to. Armed with a new awareness of what you put into your body and how it makes you feel on a superficial and cellular level, you can successfully handle any situation life throws your way without being thrown off your game. You know what your body needs now to thrive and shine. And remember, being healthy is about more than managing your weight—it's about cultivating and then embracing a lifestyle that, day-to-day, makes you feel and look your best.

WEEK 4 MOVE YOUR BODY: MODERATE EXERCISE

This week, keep up the physical intensity from last week with cardio exercise and moderate strength training. If you so desire, further intensify with high-pitch spinning, running, heavy weight training, cardio classes, and even endurance sports. These activities are a kick-butt complement to week 4 because your body should have boundless energy and fuel to support the high-intensity activities you love. If you're not feeling it, then give it a rest. Kick down the intensity. Just be sure to keep moving. Set aside regular times to utilize the fuel you're putting into your body. This is no time to lose the healthy momentum you've built over the past 28 days. Rather, now, is the perfect time to keep the fire burning!,

This Could Totally Be You:
Tons of Energy

"My business has me traveling for a living and this makes my nutritional needs a daily challenge. Juicing saves me a great deal of time, money, and worry about what sustenance I will have at my next 'stop.' I am often complimented on my skin and 'glow' and overall youthful appearance. I give the credit to juicing and healthy eating in general. It's enabled me to maintain a healthy weight and I have tons of energy, waking up with a smile each day."

—Amy E., 51, longtime juicer and artist

WEEK 4 SHOPPING LIST

This week's shopping list has it all! Refer to this all-inclusive list to prepare all of the nutrient-dense juices and whole-food recipes from the full 28-day program, and to create your own nutritional plan that you will sustain into the future with ease.

Week 4 Shopping Tip: Meal Planning

This week, it's time to test your meal-planning skills as you prepare to step away from the 28-day program and back into your everyday life, where you will be responsible for your own nutritional plan. This week, notice where you can double or triple up on recipes to portion out for snacks or meals later in the day or week. For example, if you're making hummus for the Mediterranean Medley salad, double up so you have something savory to dip veggies in throughout the week. If you're preparing salmon, bake two large pieces of fresh fish so you have extra for mixing into an egg scramble the next morning or for enjoying over a green leafy salad for a quick and easy lunch assembly. Double portions of grains to toss into salads or breakfast cereals. By preparing big batches, you cut down on your prep and cooking time and maximize your mealtime.

Fresh Produce

- Artichokes
- Arugula
- Asparagus
- Baby greens
- Beets, beet greens
- Bell pepper (green and red)
- Bok choy
- Broccoli
- Brussels sprouts
- Butter lettuce
- Cabbage (green and red)
- Carrots
- Cauliflower
- Celery
- Collard greens
- Cucumber
- Dandelion greens
- Eggplant
- Endive
- Fennel
- Green beans
- Green bell pepper
- Green garden peas
- Green leaf lettuce
- Green onion
- Jicama
- Kale
- Leeks
- Mushrooms
- Pea sprouts
- Red onion
- Romaine leaf lettuce
- Shallots
- Spinach
- Sugar snap peas
- Sweet potato
- Swiss chard
- Watercress
- Winter Squash (acorn, butternut, delicata, Hubbard, kabocha, pumpkin, spaghetti)
- Yams
- Zucchini (green and yellow)

Fresh Whole Fruit

Apples (all)

Avocados

Bananas

Berries (blackberry, blueberry, raspberry, strawberry)

Cantaloupe

Cherries

Dates

Figs

Grapes

Grapefruit

Honeydew melon

Kiwi

Lemons

Limes

Mangoes

Nectarines

Oranges

Papaya

Peaches

Pears

Pineapple

Plums

Tomatoes (any)

Watermelon

Grains

Amaranth

Barley

Brown rice and brown rice cakes and tortillas

Buckwheat

Hemp seed

Kamut

Millet

Oats (whole) and oat bran

Quinoa

Rye

Spelt

Wheat (preferably sprouted) bread and tortillas

Wheat berries

Proteins

Bacon (pork or beef, nitrate-free)

Beans (all)— black beans, butter beans, cannellini beans, chickpeas, edamame soy beans, great northern beans, kidney beans, lentils, lima beans, navy beans, pinto beans

Beef (grass-fed)

Beef jerky (nitrate-free, unsweetened)

Bison (grass-fed)

Canned salmon, sardines, or tuna (no oil or sodium)

Chicken (organic, skinless, white meat) and chicken sausage

Eggs (organic, free-range)

Lamb (grass-fed)

Lunch meat turkey, chicken, **ham** (organic, low sodium, nitrate-free)

Pork and pork sausage

Turkey (organic, oven-roasted), turkey sausage, and turkey bacon (nitrate-free)

Wild-caught fish, shellfish (see page 31 for a list of the healthiest and safest choices)

Dairy

Cow's milk, butter, cheese, yogurt, kefir (organic, unsweetened)

Goat's milk, butter, cheese, yogurt, **kefir** (organic, unsweetened)

Sheep's milk, butter, cheese, yogurt, kefir (organic, unsweetened)

Healthy Fats: Nuts, Seeds, and Butters

(Preferably unroasted, unsalted, and unsweetened)

- Almonds and almond butter
- Brazil nuts
- **Cashews and cashew butter**
- Chia seeds
- Flaxseeds
- Hazelnuts and hazelnut butter
- Macadamia nuts and macadamia butter
- Pecans
- Pine nuts
- Pumpkin seeds
- Sesame seeds
- Sunflower seeds and sunflower butter
- Tahini
- Walnuts

Fresh and Dried Herbs

Any and all! This week prepare juices and whole-food meals with your favorite dried or fresh herbs

Spices and Seasonings

Any and all! This week prepare juices and whole-food meals with your favorite dried or fresh spices and seasonings

Natural Sweeteners and non-dairy milks

- Almond milk (unsweetened)
- Cacao powder
- **Cashew milk (unsweetened)**
- Coconut milk (unsweetened)
- Coconut palm sugar
- Coconut water
- **Dark chocolate chips**
- Date sugar
- Hazelnut milk (unsweetened)
- Honey (preferably raw)
- Maple syrup
- Shredded coconut (unsweetened)
- Stevia (organic or "whole leaf")
- Vanilla extract

Essential Oils and Pantry Staples

- Apple cider vinegar
- Avocado oil
- Balsamic vinegar
- Broth, vegetable and chicken (low sodium, no yeast or sugar)
- Caffeinated coffee
- Caffeinated herbal tea
- Coconut oil
- Cold-pressed flax oil
- Decaf espresso powder
- Dijon mustard
- Extra-virgin olive oil
- Ghee (clarified butter)
- Macadamia nut oil
- Miso
- Red wine vinegar
- Tamari
- Walnut oil
- Vinegar

Remember: This week, it's not required that you crowd out any foods; just make your preferred choices, meal by meal, juice by juice. That's right—eat and drink as you would on a typical day, although don't be too surprised to discover that after 21 days of hydrating with nutrient-dense juices and eating whole-food nutrition, what's typical has changed. The foods you crave this week may be drastically different from what you were hungry for three weeks ago. You may discover that given the choice, you choose foods from the in-crowd list over others.

You seriously rock! You've just unlocked your highest health potential. Over the past 28 days you've learned how to shop for, prepare, and eat a more nutritious, balanced, and clean diet by combining fresh juice with whole-food meals and crowding out the biggest offenders to your health like added sugars, saturated fats, and processed foods. Our time together has given you just a taste of how wonderful you can look and feel for the rest of your life, with increased energy, clear skin, better sleep, fantastic focus, reduced cravings, and a more lean, fluid body. You've set the foundation for sustainable health, and now it's time for you to take all that you've learned and practiced and move forward with your beautiful life.

Completing the Suja Juice Solution is a major achievement and you should feel deservedly proud and liberated. At the same time, your newfound freedom to forge ahead and create the lifestyle of your individual choosing means you're 100 percent responsible for keeping yourself on track. This can be a challenge, and we both know this well, which is why before sending you on your way, we'd like to share our best solutions for staying on the lifelong path toward optimal health and wellness when the demands of real life get in the way.

CHAPTER 11

The SUJA LIFESTYLE

KEEP JUICING

Nutrient-dense juice just has a magical way of bringing out your inner radiance. So continue to drink up and shine! Juice will keep you sufficiently hydrated with water, along with essential nutrients, minerals, and electrolytes. This is so important. Second, juicing is an efficient way to get a daily dose of garden-fresh greens. Juicing removes the fiber from fruits and veggies, so your body has less work to do in breaking them down, allowing you to quickly access and assimilate their vital nutrients and enzymes. One juice easily packs multiple servings of fresh, organic produce into one glass. Finally, drinking juice before a meal will help satiate you and curb unhealthy cravings and mindless snacking. Did you know that hunger is often confused with thirst? Juice will fill you up for longer between meals and help you to maintain a healthy weight.

EAT AND PREPARE POWER-FOOD MEALS

We hope you've cultivated a new appreciation for fresh, colorful foods over the past 28 days, and lost your taste for processed junky foods that can easily slow you down, zap your energy, and exacerbate stress. Healthy habits begin at the grocery store, so continue to power up with seasonal and organic produce. When you ensure that you're putting quality fuel into your body, you're much better equipped to handle the challenges life throws your way. Also, continue to take time to plan and prepare your meals. This way, you can be 100 percent in control of what you're putting into your body. Cooking connects you to your food; it can also be very therapeutic, and a wonderfully creative way to manage stress.

START THE DAY OFF RIGHT

Mornings can be rushed and hectic, but you only set yourself up for an inevitable downslide if you don't take the time to nourish your body well before heading out the door. If you don't feel your best, you won't look or perform at your best. It's that simple, so at the very least start your morning by slugging a mug of warm water with a squeeze of lemon and a pinch of cayenne to wake up your digestive tract, stimulate your liver (your main detoxifying organ), and give you an energy boost. This hydrating morning tonic will get you going. Although, it will only get you so far. You still need to also eat nourishing foods to fuel your activities and maintain your physical energy, mental awareness, and focus throughout the day. If sitting down to breakfast is just not going to happen for you, make it a habit to grab food 'n' go.

KEEP MOVING

Continue to match your activity level with the amount of juice and whole-food nutrition you're consuming daily, and remember that not every day calls for a major workout. Often a 30-minute brisk walk or a gentle yoga class is enough to reset and reenergize you. Movement will continue to play a major role in your healthy weight management and efficient digestion, and also to help reduce stress hormones, release tension, and balance your energy.

GET A GOOD NIGHT'S REST

If you aren't sleeping well, you'll be much less equipped to take on life's inevitable stresses, and you'll have far less willpower and motivation to make healthy choices if you're tired. Missing sleep can also impair cellular and cognitive function—in other words, zap your brainpower and make you sick. Furthermore, poor sleep has been linked to numerous health issues like weight gain, depression, and high blood pressure. So get your ZZZZs. It's imperative to your physical and mental health that your body have the opportunity to rest and recover.

WATCH THE BOOZE

Who doesn't love a happy hour? But if you aren't watching it, you can easily consume hundreds of empty calories before the second round. To avoid this, skip the cream-based and sugary mixed drinks. Opt for low-calorie mixers like soda water and citrus instead, or shake up your own low-glycemic spirits and cocktails. For inspiration check out our selection of sip-worthy spirits in chapter 16.

THINK BEFORE YOU EAT

You've reset your body to a cleaner, more balanced state, and eating less-than-healthy foods can easily upset that balance you've worked so hard to set in place. Moving forward, continue the practice of mindful nutrition. Before preparing or ordering a meal, give careful consideration to what foods will both physically and mentally serve you the best, and then pay attention to your food as you're eating it. Did you know that mindless eating often leads to feelings of dissatisfaction and subsequent overeating? So take notice of the smells, tastes, and textures of the food you're putting into your body. You'll enjoy it much more and you'll likely only eat the amount that your body truly needs. With daily repletion, mindful eating will become an almost mindless activity.

CLEAN HOUSE

If you're the parent of a toddler, you take steps to childproof your home. You put locks on the doors and gates on the stairs to keep your child safe. In a similar way, if you want to protect your health, why not junk-proof your home? We're not suggesting you put locks on your cabinets or bars in front of your fridge, but do take steps to create a healthy environment for yourself that is conducive to the person you want to be. Meaning—if you want to be your best-looking and -feeling self, bring only the healthiest foods and ingredients into your home—vibrant fresh produce, juicy fruits, fresh omega-3-rich fish, organic grass-fed meat, vitamin-packed whole grains, and healthy fats.

TRAVEL SMART

Expect that when traveling, your healthy food and juice options may be limited. Still, no one wants to ruin a trip sweating over every meal, so aim to strike a healthy balance between enjoying yourself and taking care of yourself. In other words—have your fun *in moderation.*

- **Pack healthy foods.** Instead of eating four bags of salted peanuts or bringing aboard a pre-packaged ham-and-cheese sandwich from the airport, pack your favorite healthy snacks in your carry-on bag. On longer flights, pack a healthy meal in a soft cooler. You'll be so glad you did (and the person sitting next to you will wish they did too).

- **Shop locally for fresh foods.** Purchase fruits and veggies at the grocery store or corner market nearest to your hotel and stash them in the mini fridge. This will curb any temptation that might take hold to gobble the $10 M&M's from the mini bar.

- **Pick your restaurants ahead of time.** Do a little research. Ask around, search online reviews, or reference your favorite restaurant-finder apps to discover the healthiest dining options in the city you're traveling or neighborhood you're staying *before* hunger strikes.

EVERY MEAL IS A NEW BEGINNING

Day-to-day, you won't always make the healthiest choices, and that's okay. A single slipup at your best friend's bachelorette party doesn't mean defeat—nor does it give you permission to go totally off the rails and order an extra-large pizza at midnight. Don't listen to the voice in your head that tries to make you feel bad about yourself. Remember, you're human and the path forward is never a straight line. Curves, dips, and even potholes are the way you get from where you are now to where you want to be. If critical thoughts sneak in, remind yourself of everything you've accomplished over the past 28 days, and then get out of your head. Go for a brisk 20-minute walk, take a yoga class, or simply breathe deeply for 5 minutes, then tell yourself, "Every meal is a new beginning."

STAY CONNECTED

Continue to check in and stay connected with family members, friends, and colleagues who are also committed to sustaining a healthy lifestyle. Be willing to share your weak moments, challenges, and triumphs. Take these opportunities to set new fitness and nutrition goals together and to recommit to long-term health. These supportive relationships will continue to serve as an important reminder of all you have accomplished and to give you strength when you most need it.

REPEAT THE SUJA JUICE SOLUTION AS NEEDED

If at any time you feel like you need some extra motivation to get "healthy"—maybe you've just returned from an indulgent vacation, or work stress is sabotaging your best nutritional efforts—you may always return to the program to quickly reset your body in 7 days. It's not necessary to repeat all 28 days (though you're welcome to); you'll likely only need a short reset. Recommit yourself to 7 days of juice hydration and whole-food nutrition to flush out excess waste and water weight, curb cravings, boost energy and focus, and regain a healthy equilibrium. While we're firm believers in sustainable health, we certainly don't advocate *dieting* for the rest of your life. Ugh—where's the fun in that? Instead, you can easily maintain your optimal health by relying on your new level of awareness of what foods best nourish, satisfy, and energize you. In addition to nourishing yourself well, spend time engaging in other activities that fill and light you up. People who live with humor and passion are often the healthiest and happiest. Be one of them!

Part 3

RECIPES

Now for the fun part—the recipes! Simple, beautiful, healthful, and delicious. They're the shining stars of this program, and we're so excited to share them with you. We hope that you enjoy them as much as we do and make them your own as you experience the excitement and gratification of preparing whole-food meals that do your mind and body good. The Suja Juice Solution is not about deprivation—far from it—and the recipes in these chapters are delicious proof of that. Living the Suja lifestyle means enjoying the food you eat and knowing that it nourishes your body. When you prepare your own food, you know exactly what you're eating, and you can choose ingredients that make you feel satisfied on every level. Since we eat with our eyes first, we believe that it's important to prepare food that aesthetically pleases. Next comes health. We eat to provide our body with the nutrients it needs to function at its highest level, and finally we eat for pleasure—to enjoy and savor real, whole food that tastes delicious. In the pages ahead, we've included over 75 recipes for morning, midday, and early-evening meals, along with grab 'n' go snack ideas, sin-free sweets, and everything you need to know to

CHAPTER 12

WEEK 1: RESET

Recipes + shopping guide

make your own juices, elixirs, and tonics at home. We've even included 30-plus bonus hydration recipes for when you're craving something extra juicy. We hope you find that these recipes make it a true pleasure to follow the Suja Juice Solution.

Before you get juicing and cooking, here are a few notes to keep in mind:

- **Portions.** Unless otherwise noted, all recipes make one serving. Feel free to double or triple any of the meal recipes if you're feeding more than just yourself, or if you prefer to make larger batches for multiple meals. Juice recipes can easily be doubled, too, to satisfy your midday and early-evening hydration needs.

- **Seasoning.** Feel free to add salt, pepper, fresh lemon juice, and any herbs and spices of your liking to all dishes to enhance flavor. Stevia can also be added to all juice recipes for additional sweetness.

- **Juice prep.** If you don't have time to fire up the juicer, we've simplified each of the juice recipes into Juice Bar Blends so that you can easily order them at your local juice bar to grab 'n' go. For blender users, we've made each of the juices blender-friendly by adding a few key ingredients to make it a smoothie.

A Note from the Juice Chef

"My mantra regarding food has always been—if it tastes good, then stop overthinking it and *just eat it!* The best dishes make you *feel good*—physically and mentally—and they tend to be the ones comprised of the cleanest and freshest ingredients. What I love about cooking and creating original juice recipes for Suja is that I get to introduce fruit and vegetable combinations to people that they've probably never tried before, most often because they're convinced they won't like them. I've met a lot of people who have an automatic aversion to kale and collards, beets and celery, but once they can get past their reluctance and that barrier to give them a try, they're almost always blown away by the taste and by how awesome they make you feel."

—Bryan Riblett, CIA graduate,
VP of commercialization,
and head of innovation for Suja

WEEK 1 RECIPES

Week 1 Recipes at a Glance

JUICES

Sweet and Simple

Spa Kick

Leafy Grapefruit Kick

Fennel and Friends

MORNING MEALS

Charged-Up Chia Pudding

Under the Sea Spinach Omelet

Sunrise Grapefruit and Avocado Salad

MIDDAY MEALS

Lentil Love Salad

Avocado Tuna Collard Roll

Kale-ifornia Salad

EARLY-EVENING MEALS

Simply Salmon

Zesty Zucchini Basil Soup

Totally Guacamoly Tacos

Morning Juice Hydration

Both juice recipes make 16 ounces.

Sweet and Simple

3 lemons, peeled

2 tablespoons apple cider vinegar

Pinch of cayenne

Stevia, to taste

12 ounces water

Juice the lemons and stir in the other ingredients.

JUICE BAR BLEND: Lemon, water.

Tip: Carry stevia packets with you for some extra sweetness when the sweetener is unavailable at your local juice bar.

Spa Kick

3 medium cucumbers (with skins)

1 cup watercress (loosely packed)

1 inch raw unpeeled gingerroot

2 lemons, peeled

Stevia (optional), to taste

Juice all the ingredients and stir in the stevia if desired.

JUICE BAR BLEND: Cucumber, celery, lemon, ginger.

BLENDER RECIPE: Replace two of the cucumbers with 6 ounces coconut water. Squeeze the lemons by hand and peel and grate the ginger before blending until smooth.

> ➤ *SPOTLIGHT ON LEMON*
> Lemon juice is a vitamin-C-rich alkaline-forming food that helps wake up the body by stimulating tummy acids and natural enzymes. Drinking lemon juice first thing in the morning provides the body with a good dose of cleansing power, helping to flush out waste and promote elimination.

Morning Meals

Charged-Up Chia Pudding

. . . .

NOTE: This is a make-the-night-before recipe. Planning ahead is necessary.

1 cup unsweetened almond or coconut milk

¼ cup chia seeds

1 tablespoon ground flaxseeds

Pinch of cinnamon, to taste

Stevia, to taste

1 tablespoon shredded coconut (unsweetened)

Before bed, place the almond milk, chia seeds, flaxseeds, cinnamon, and stevia in a bowl (or, our personal preference, a mason jar). Stir the ingredients together really well, making sure the chia is evenly distributed and not clumping. Place the bowl or jar in the fridge, allowing it to gel up to a thick, pudding-like consistency overnight. In the morning, remove the mixture to a bowl, add the shredded coconut on top for garnish, and dig in.

► *SPOTLIGHT ON CHIA SEEDS*

We love chia seeds because they're so good for you and so fun to eat! These little black seeds are a tremendous source of fiber and omega-3 fatty acids. Also, these little guys contain iron, calcium, zinc, and antioxidants, and can help hydrate the body because they carry liquid when soaked. One of the most unique qualities of chia seeds is their ability to absorb liquid then gel up and thicken into a pudding-like consistency. Chia puddings made with water or non-dairy milk are a great way to pack healthy ingredients into a simple meal. Just a 1-ounce serving of chia has approximately 11 grams of dietary fiber, or a third of the recommended daily intake for adults.

Under the Sea Spinach Omelet

· · · · · · · · · · · · · · · · ·

2 eggs

Pinch of sea salt, to taste

Pinch of black pepper, to taste

1/4 teaspoon garlic powder

2 teaspoons coconut oil or ghee

1/2 large Portobello mushroom

1 cup spinach

2–3 pieces dulse seaweed, chopped

In a small bowl, whisk together the eggs, sea salt, black pepper, and garlic powder. Set the mixture aside. Place a skillet over medium heat and add the coconut oil or ghee, allowing it to heat up. While this happens, chop the Portobello mushroom into strips and roughly chop the spinach into smaller pieces. When the oil or ghee is heated, pour the egg mixture into the skillet and allow it to cook for a minute or two until the bottom is golden brown. Add the spinach, dulse, and mushroom on one side of the omelet. With a spatula, flip the other side over the filling and turn the heat to low, letting the whole thing cook for another minute or two. Transfer to a plate and enjoy while hot.

Sunrise Grapefruit and Avocado Salad

· · · · · · · · · · · · · · · · ·

1 ruby red grapefruit

1/2 avocado, cubed

1/2 Persian cucumber, cubed, or 1 cup cubed jicama

Cinnamon, to taste

Stevia (optional)

To segment the grapefruit, cut the top and bottom off so it stands upright on a cutting board. Using a knife, slice from the top to the bottom down the length of the grapefruit along the flesh, removing the peel and white pith. When this is completed on all sides, hold the grapefruit on its side over a bowl with your hand and cut along the white membrane lines into the center of the fruit, yielding V-shaped segments of grapefruit. Set the center and membrane scraps aside. Gently halve the grapefruit segments and place them in a bowl. Add the avocado to the bowl. Take the grapefruit membrane scraps and squeeze over the salad. Add the cinnamon and stevia, if desired, and mix everything together well.

VARIATION: Instead of cinnamon, use cayenne and sea salt for a savory twist.

Midday and Early-Evening Juices

Both juice recipes make 16 ounces.

Leafy Grapefruit Kick

. . . .

1 medium cucumber (with skin)

3 stalks celery

¼ head romaine lettuce

¼ head green leaf lettuce

2 leaves lacinato kale

4 sprigs parsley

2 sprigs mint

½ grapefruit, peeled

1 inch unpeeled gingerroot

Juice all the ingredients.

JUICE BAR BLEND: Cucumber, celery, kale, parsley, grapefruit, ginger.

BLENDER RECIPE: Peel the grapefruit and remove the rind. Replace half of the cucumber with 6 ounces coconut water. Chop all greens and herbs, and peel and grate the ginger before blending until smooth.

Fennel and Friends

· · · · · · · · · · · · · · · · · ·

2 medium cucumbers (with skins)

2 stalks celery

2 leaves lacinato kale

¼ head green leaf lettuce

2 collard greens leaves

½ cup spinach

2 lemons, peeled

½ bulb fennel

Juice all the ingredients.

JUICE BAR BLEND: Cucumber, celery, spinach, kale, lemon, ginger.

BLENDER RECIPE: Replace one of the cucumbers with 6 ounces coconut water, and add the juice of one additional freshly squeezed lemon. Chop all greens before tossing into the blender. Blend until smooth.

> ➤ *SPOTLIGHT ON CUCUMBER*
> Cucumbers are a wonderful detoxifying food because they contain a lot of natural hydration. The water content of cucumbers makes them highly effective in helping flush out unwanted waste as it's released from the cells and tissues. The H$_2$O in cucumbers contains electrolytes to restore and balance the fluid levels in the body. Enjoy these hydrating, antioxidant-dense cucumber and super-green drinks for a mega dose of refreshing nutrition.

Midday Meals

Lentil Love Salad

· · · · · · · · · · · · · · · · · ·

⅓ cup home-cooked or canned lentils

2 tablespoons diced red onion

1 small Roma tomato, diced

½ clove garlic, minced

2 teaspoons olive oil

Juice of ½ lemon

½ teaspoon cumin

Sea salt, to taste

2–3 cups baby greens

Drain and rinse a can of lentils or use fresh lentils prepared by simmering in water over the stovetop for 20 to 30 minutes. Measure out ⅓ cup and add the lentils to a small bowl. Add the red onion, tomato, and garlic to the bowl, then the olive oil, lemon juice, cumin, and sea salt to taste. Mix the salad together well until all the ingredients are well combined. Place a bed of baby greens on a plate and spoon the salad on top. The greens need no additional dressing because the lentils are dressed!

Tip: Make a big batch of lentils at the beginning of the week and store them in an airtight container in the fridge. This makes throwing this salad together, along with the Totally Guacamoly Tacos (page 142), a cinch throughout the week.

➤ *SPOTLIGHT ON LENTILS*

Fall in love with lentils! They are the one and only legume on the in-crowd list this week. Lentils are the exception because their protein-to-carb ratio is better balanced than other legumes like black, kidney, or garbanzo beans. They'll fill you up and add heartiness to meatless meals. They're also extremely high in soluble fiber that helps your body manage blood sugar levels.

Avocado Tuna Collard Roll

. . . .

1 small can chunk light tuna in water (substitute canned salmon)

¼ red bell pepper, diced

¼ avocado

1 tablespoon Dijon mustard

1 large collard leaf

3–4 pea sprouts

Drain the can of tuna and use a fork to break it up in a bowl. Add the bell pepper and, using the fork, mash the avocado and Dijon into the mixture until it is creamy and well combined.

Lay out the collard leaf and remove the tough stem by slicing along each side of it. Spoon the tuna mixture onto one side of the collard leaf in the center and place the pea sprouts on top. Fold the opposite side over the filling and roll the collard leaf up like a burrito. Cut into sushi rolls and enjoy!

Kale-ifornia Salad

. . . .

1 head kale, de-stemmed

½ red onion, diced

1 whole avocado, cubed

1½ tablespoons tamari

2 tablespoons Dijon mustard

1 tablespoon garlic powder

1 pint cherry tomatoes

Wash the kale and finely chop it using a good knife. Place the kale in a bowl. Add the red onion, avocado, tamari, Dijon, and garlic powder to the bowl. Using your hands, massage all of the ingredients together for 2 to 3 minutes, allowing the kale to soften and the avocado to form a creamy dressing with the tamari and Dijon. Halve the cherry tomatoes and gently toss them into the salad.

Makes 2 servings

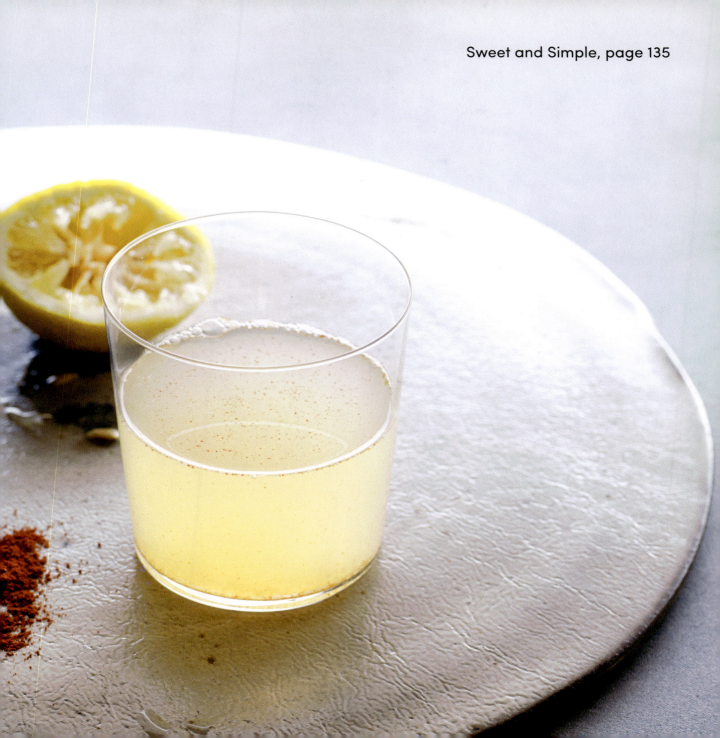
Sweet and Simple, page 135

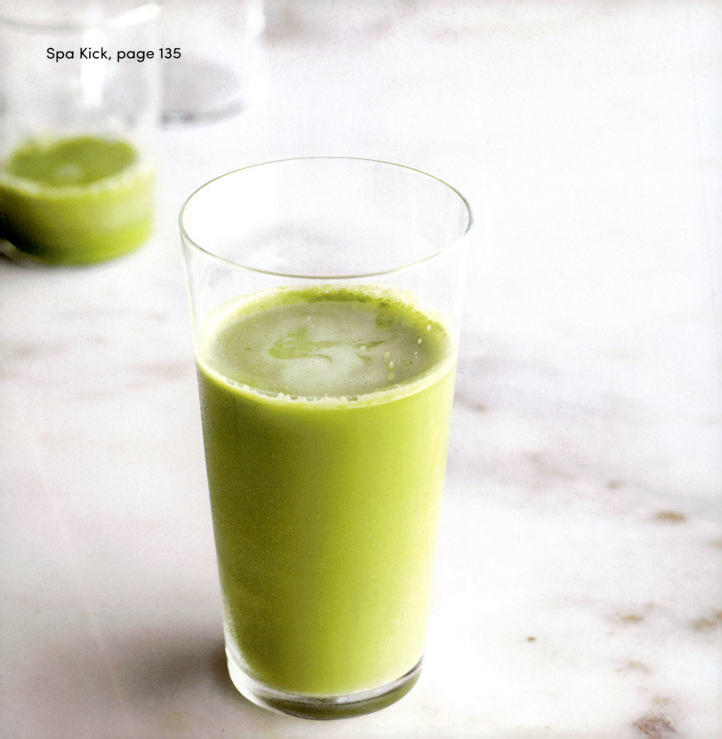

Spa Kick, page 135

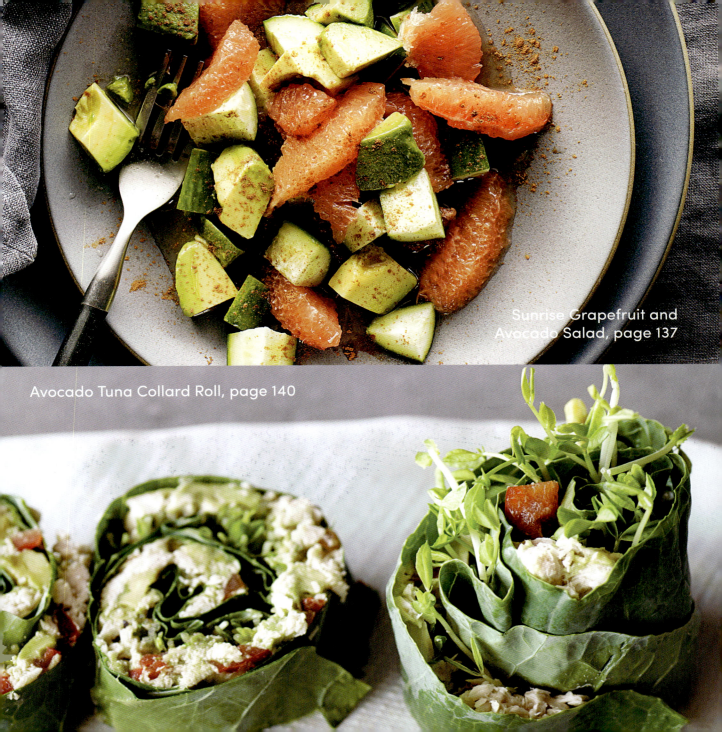

Sunrise Grapefruit and Avocado Salad, page 137

Avocado Tuna Collard Roll, page 140

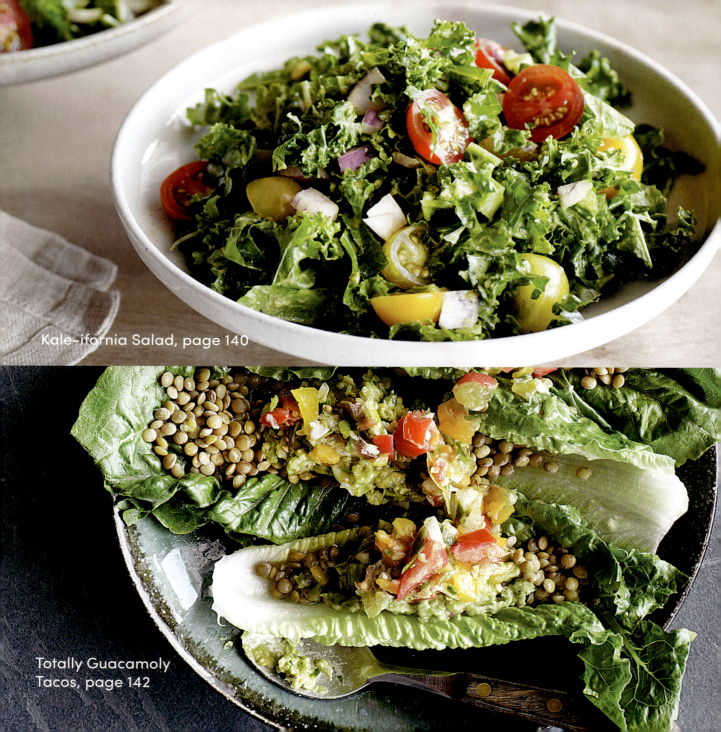

Kale–ifornia Salad, page 140

Totally Guacamoly
Tacos, page 142

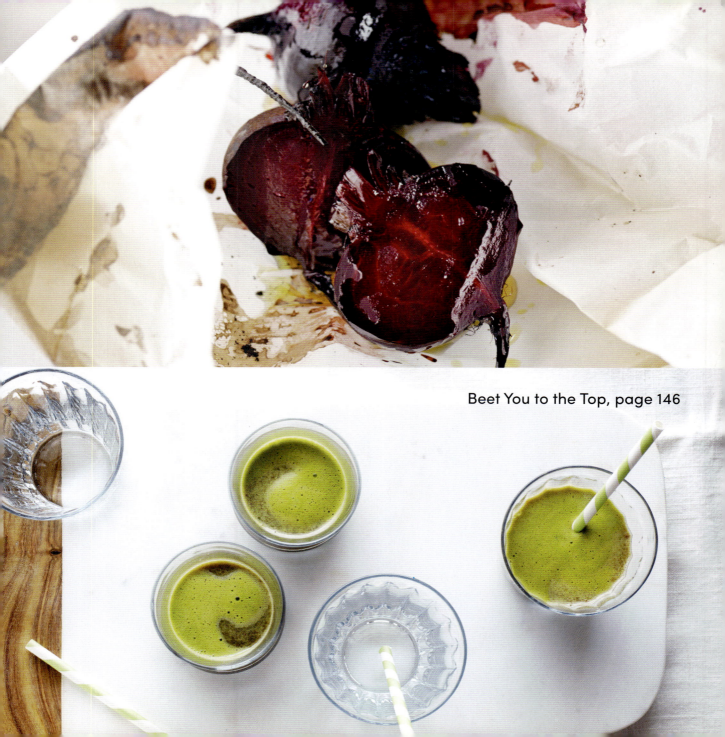

Beet You to the Top, page 146

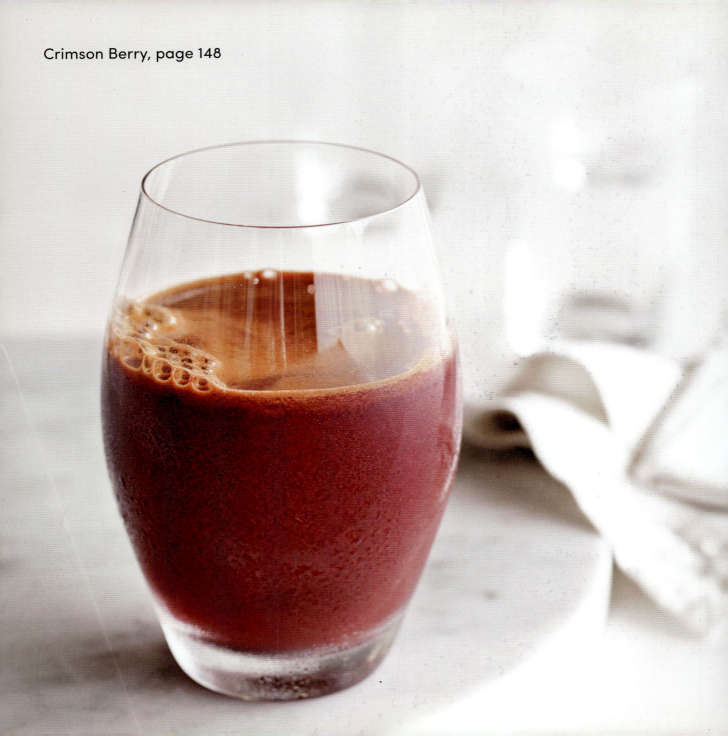

Crimson Berry, page 148

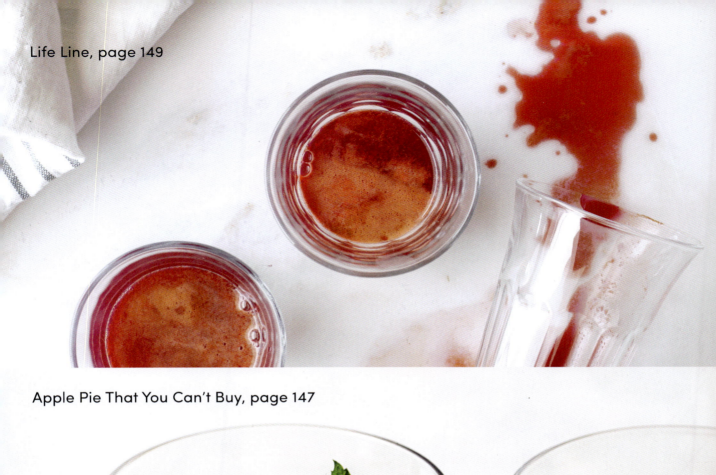

Life Line, page 149

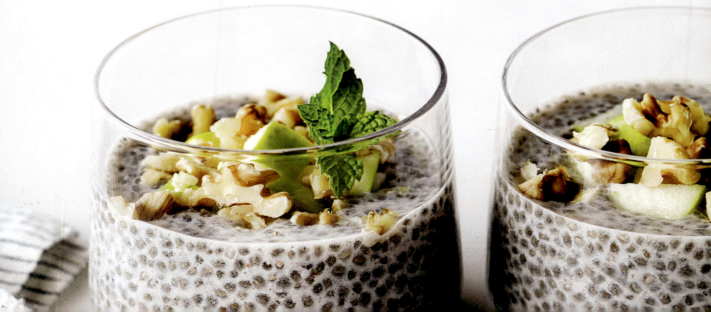

Apple Pie That You Can't Buy, page 147

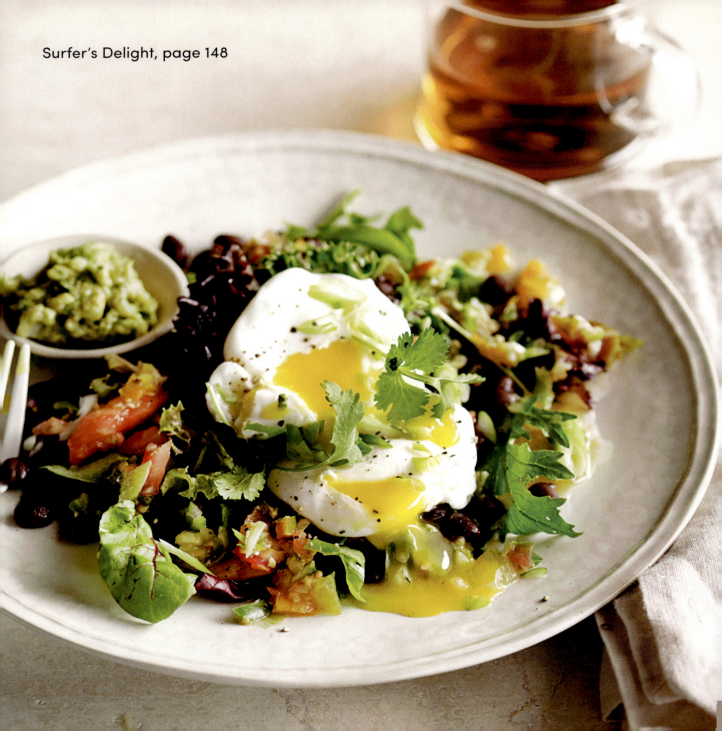

Surfer's Delight, page 148

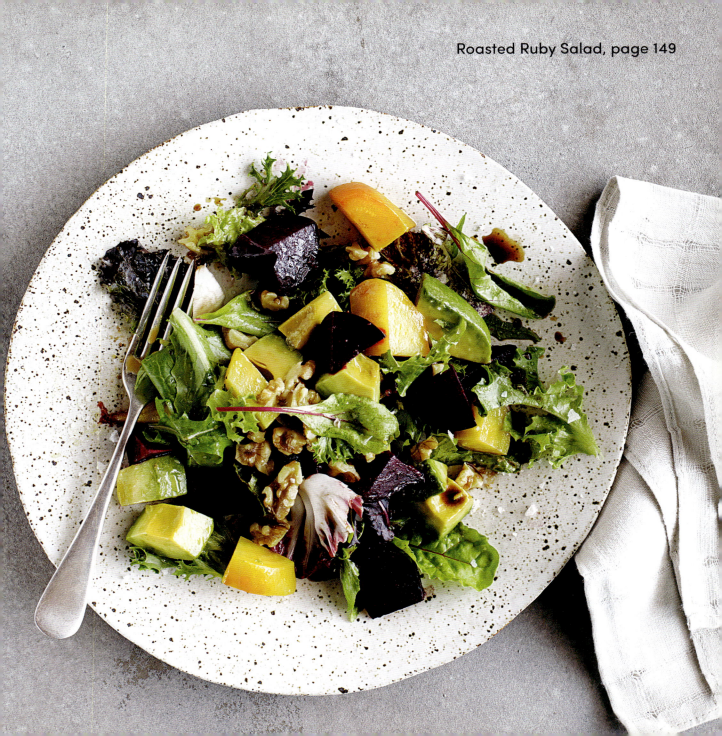

Roasted Ruby Salad, page 149

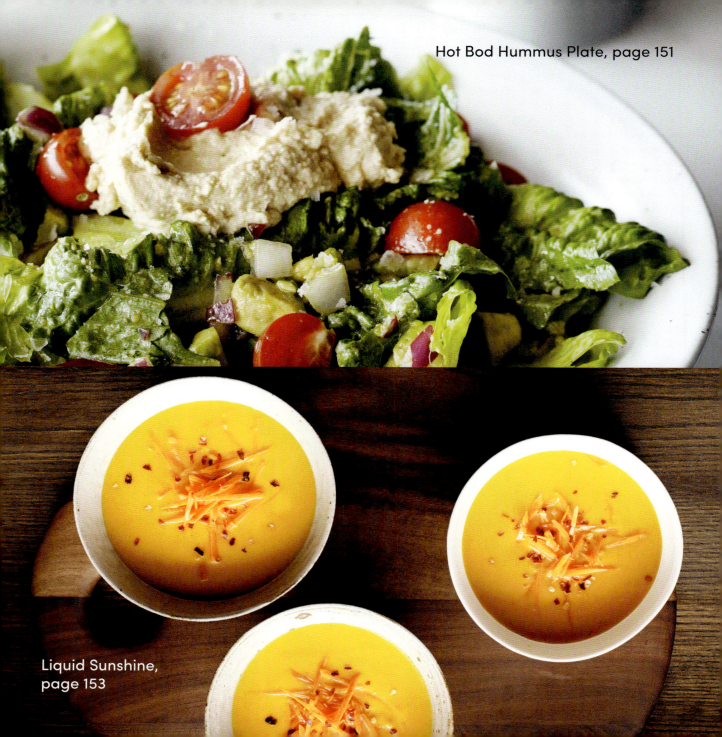

Hot Bod Hummus Plate, page 151

Liquid Sunshine,
page 153

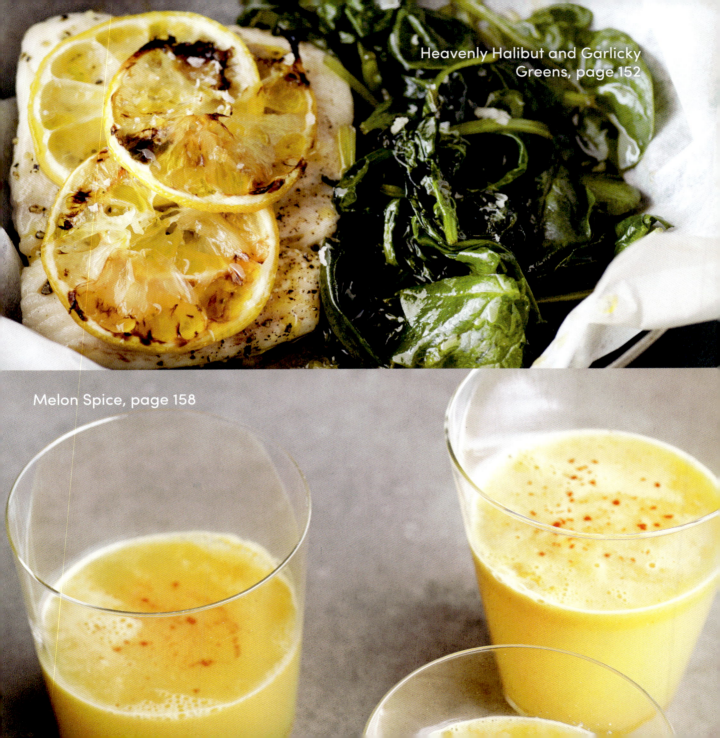

Heavenly Halibut and Garlicky
Greens, page 152

Melon Spice, page 158

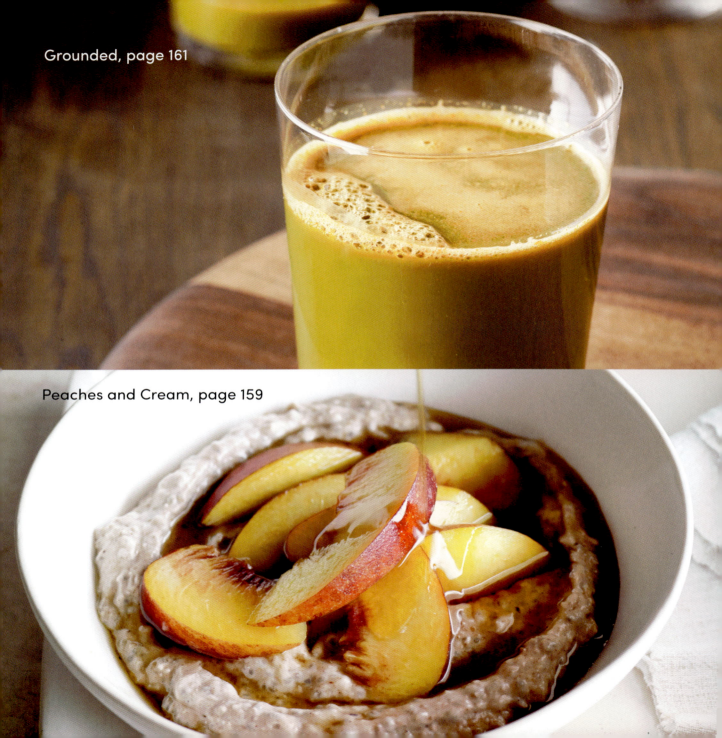

Grounded, page 161

Peaches and Cream, page 159

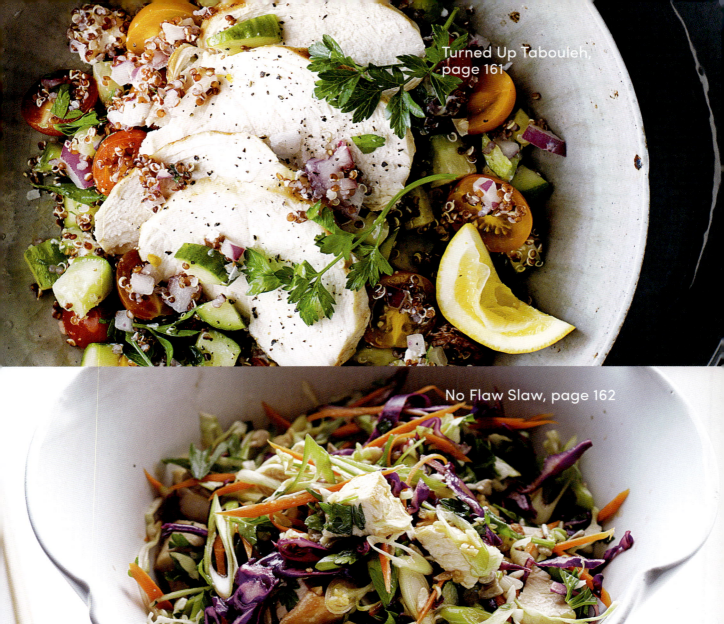

Turned Up Tabouleh, page 161

No Flaw Slaw, page 162

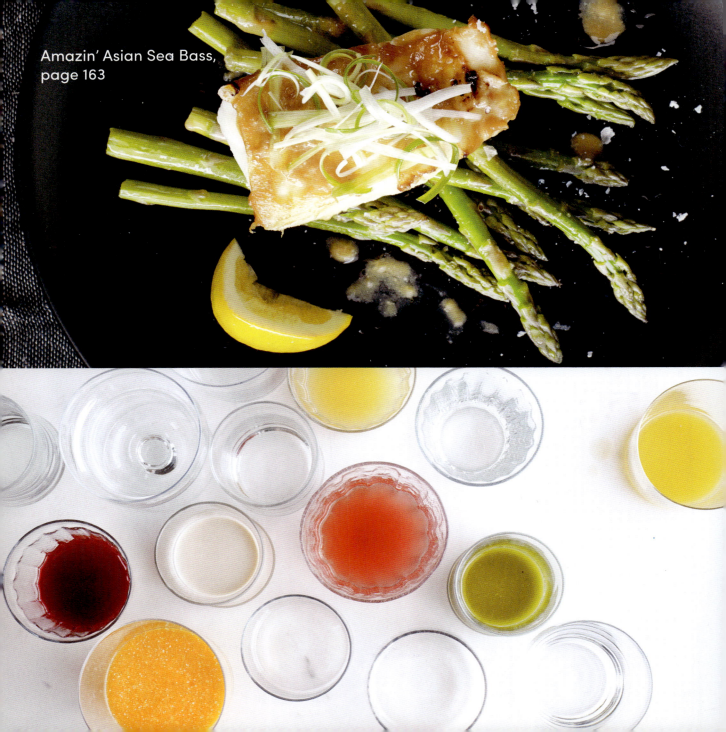

Amazin' Asian Sea Bass,
page 163

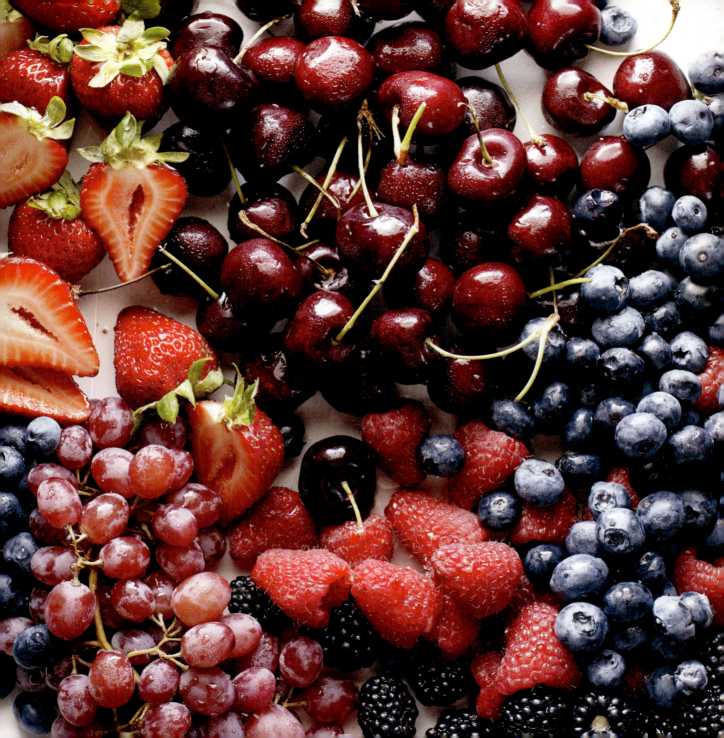

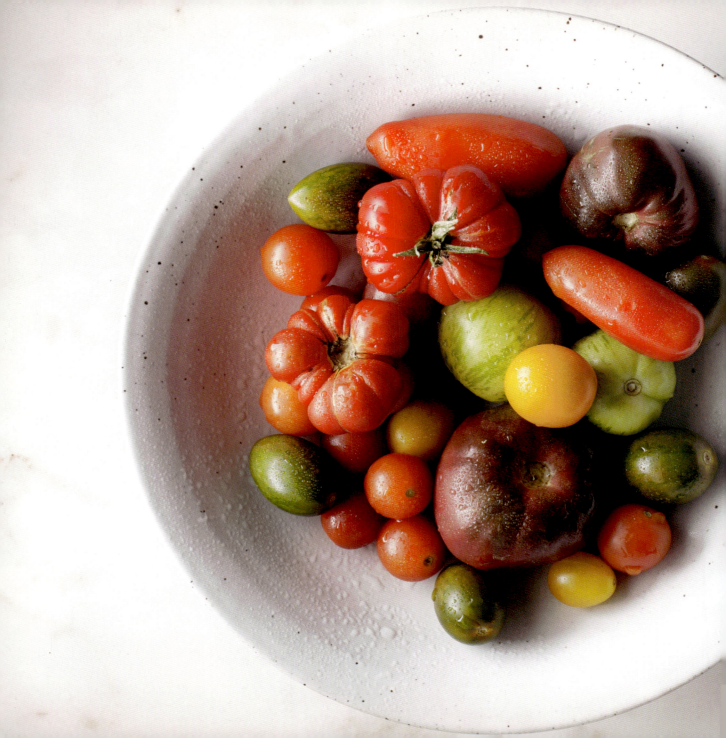

Early-Evening Meals

Simply Salmon

· · · · · · · · · · · · · · · ·

1 (4-ounce) salmon fillet (or skinless chicken breast)

1 teaspoon sea salt

$\frac{1}{2}$ teaspoon black pepper

2 teaspoons chopped fresh rosemary

2 teaspoons minced fresh garlic

1–2 cups raw broccoli florets

Juice of $\frac{1}{2}$ lemon

Preheat the oven to 400°F and line a baking sheet with parchment paper. Place the salmon on the baking sheet and sprinkle with the sea salt, black pepper, rosemary, and garlic. Bake the salmon for 12 to 18 minutes, depending on how cooked you prefer your fish. While the salmon bakes, place a steamer basket over a saucepan with water and bring to a boil. Place the broccoli in the steamer basket and put the lid on. Allow it to steam for 4 to 6 minutes, until the broccoli is softened but still has some crunch. Place the salmon and broccoli on a plate. Squeeze the juice of half a lemon over the broccoli and sprinkle with sea salt to taste.

Zesty Zucchini Basil Soup

· · · · · · · · · · · · · · · ·

1 cup freshly squeezed orange juice

$\frac{1}{2}$ cup filtered water

1 tablespoon lemon juice

$1\frac{1}{2}$ cups chopped zucchini

$\frac{3}{4}$ avocado

3 slices serrano chile (optional)

10 basil leaves

1 clove garlic

1 cup spinach

2 teaspoons grated ginger

Sea salt, to taste

Chopped green onion, for topping

This is an easy soup to make because the blender does most of the work for you! Add the liquids to the blender first—orange juice, water, and lemon juice. Roughly chop the zucchini, avocado, serrano, basil, garlic, and spinach and add them to the blender. Using a microplane, grate the ginger and add it with the sea salt to the blender. Blend all the ingredients until completely smooth and well combined. Pour the soup into a bowl and garnish with chopped green onion. Enjoy warm if you're making in advance or room temperature if you're dining immediately.

Makes 2 servings

Totally Guacamoly Tacos

. . . .

3 large romaine leaves

½ cup home-cooked or canned lentils

⅓ cup guacamole (see below)

¼ cup salsa (see below)

GUACAMOLE

2 ripe avocados

2 tablespoons chopped cilantro or flat-leaf parsley

1 clove garlic

2 tablespoons diced red onion

1 tablespoon lime juice

Sea salt, to taste

SALSA

3 whole vine-ripened or Roma tomatoes— if heirloom varieties are available to you, try these for a gorgeous rainbow of colors!

2 tablespoons chopped cilantro or flat-leaf parsley

1 small onion

4 green onions

1 seeded serrano chile (optional)

2 cloves garlic

Juice of 1 lime

Sea salt, to taste

Assemble the base of the tacos by placing the romaine leaves on a plate. Drain a can of lentils or use fresh by simmering over the stovetop for 20 to 30 minutes. Add them to the center of the romaine leaves, evenly distributed among the three.

Make the guacamole by roughly chopping the avocados, cilantro, garlic, and red onion and adding them to the food processor. Squeeze in the lime juice and sprinkle in sea salt to taste. Pulse the guacamole to your desired consistency—chunky or smooth—and scoop on top of the lentils.

Make the salsa by roughly chopping the tomatoes, cilantro, red onion, green onions, serrano chile, and garlic and adding them to the food processor. Squeeze in the lime juice and sprinkle in sea salt to taste. Pulse the salsa to your desired consistency and scoop on top of the tacos.

Week 1 Create-Your-Own Meals

This week, you're invited to create your own morning, midday, and early-evening meals from the charts below by combining ingredients from each column.

Meat Eater's Meal

PROTEIN	FRESH GREEN VEGGIES	HEALTHY FATS
4 ounces lean protein	Unlimited	1 tablespoon healthy oil, or 2 tablespoons nuts, or ⅓ avocado

Vegetarian Meal

PROTEIN	FRESH GREEN VEGGIES	HEALTHY FATS
¾ cup cooked lentils	Unlimited	1 tablespoon healthy oil, or 2 tablespoons nuts, or ⅓ avocado

WEEK 1 SHOPPING LIST

Your week 1 shopping list includes all the ingredients you'll need over the next 7 days to create the reset juices and whole-food recipes. For a complete list of all the foods and ingredients that make the "In Crowd" this week, refer back to chapter 7, page 72. Throughout the program, you're welcome to create your own nutritious and delicious dishes from the comprehensive list of week 1 "In Crowd" foods. It's all about getting creative!

Fresh Produce

Baby greens

Broccoli

Celery

Collard greens

Cucumber

Fennel

Green leaf lettuce

Green onion

Jicama

Kale (Jacinto)

Pea sprouts

Portobello mushrooms

Red bell pepper

Red onion

Romaine leaf lettuce

Spinach

Watercress

Zucchini (green and yellow)

Fresh Whole Fruit

Avocados

Grapefruit

Lemons

Limes

Oranges (in soup only)

Tomatoes (Roma, cherry)

Proteins

Canned salmon, sardines, or tuna (no oil or sodium)

Chicken (organic, skinless, white meat)

Eggs (organic, free-range)

Lentils

Wild-caught salmon

Healthy Fats: Nuts and Seeds

(Preferably unroasted, unsalted)

Chia seeds

Flaxseeds

Fresh and Dried Herbs

This week prepare juices and whole-food meals with dried or fresh:

Basil

Cilantro

Dulse seaweed

Fennel

Gingerroot, ginger

Mint

Parsley (flat-leaf)

Rosemary

Spices and Seasonings

This week prepare juices and whole-food meals with dried or fresh:

Black pepper

Cayenne pepper

Cinnamon

Cumin

Garlic, garlic powder

Sea salt

Serrano chile

Natural Sweeteners and Non-Dairy Milk

Almond milk (unsweetened)

Coconut milk (unsweetened)

Coconut water (unsweetened)

Shredded coconut (unsweetened)

Stevia (organic or "whole leaf")

Essential Oils and Pantry Staples

Apple cider vinegar

Coconut oil

Dijon mustard

Extra-virgin olive oil

Ghee (clarified butter)

Tamari (gluten-free soy sauce)

Week 2 Recipes at a Glance

JUICES

Beet You to the Top

Balance

Crimson Berry

Life Line

MORNING MEALS

Apple Pie That You Can't Buy

Sweet Potato Perfection

Surfer's Delight

MIDDAY MEALS

Roasted Ruby Salad

San Diego Sando

Hot Bod Hummus Plate

EARLY-EVENING MEALS

Heavenly Halibut and Garlicky Greens

Kale-ifornia Salad 2.0

Liquid Sunshine

CHAPTER 13

WEEK 2: REINFORCE

Recipes + shopping guide

Morning Juice Hydration

Both juice recipes make 16 ounces.

Beet You to the Top

. . . .

2 Granny Smith apples

1/4 whole pineapple, peeled and cored

1 medium cucumber (with skin)

1/2 cup beet tops

1/2 cup dandelion greens

1 inch unpeeled gingerroot

Juice all the ingredients.

JUICE BAR BLEND: Apple, pineapple, cucumber, spinach, ginger.

BLENDER RECIPE: Chop all of the ingredients into small pieces for easier blending. Reduce the number of apples to one. Peel and grate the ginger, add 6 ounces coconut water to the mix, and blend all the ingredients together.

Balance

. . . .

2 Granny Smith apples

1 medium cucumber (with skin)

2 limes, peeled

1/2 inch unpeeled gingerroot

1/2 teaspoon ground turmeric

1 tablespoon apple cider vinegar

Stevia, to taste (optional)

Juice the apples, cucumber, limes, gingerroot, and turmeric. Stir in the apple cider vinegar and add stevia if needed.

JUICE BAR BLEND: Apple, cucumber, lemon, ginger.

BLENDER RECIPE: Substitute 6 ounces of pre-pressed apple juice (available at any health food store or juice shop) for the raw apples. Squeeze the lime juice by hand, chop the cucumber into small pieces, and peel and grate the ginger before blending.

> ➤ *SPOTLIGHT ON GREEN APPLE*
> Green apples are lower in sugar content than red or pink apples, and their natural tartness adds a refreshing bite to your morning green juice. Apple skins contain pectin, a soluble fiber that in combination with the enzymes and nutrients present in the apple flesh can help to lower blood sugar levels and promote healthy bacteria in the digestive tract.

Morning Meals

Apple Pie That You Can't Buy

· · · · · · · · · · · · · · ·

NOTE: This is a make-the-night-before recipe. Planning ahead is necessary.

1 cup unsweetened almond or coconut milk

¼ cup chia seeds

1 Granny Smith apple, chopped

Pinch of cinnamon, to taste

Pinch of nutmeg, to taste

Pinch of cardamom, to taste

Stevia, to taste

1 tablespoon chopped walnuts

1 sprig mint, for garnish

Before bed, place the almond milk, chia seeds, cinnamon, nutmeg, cardamom, and stevia in a bowl or mason jar. Stir the ingredients together really well, making sure the chia seeds are evenly distributed and not clumping. Place the bowl or jar in the fridge, allowing the mixture to gel up to a thick, pudding-like consistency overnight. In the morning, remove the mixture to a bowl and add the chopped apple and walnuts on top. Add a sprig of mint for garnish.

Sweet Potato Perfection

· · · · · · · · · · · · · · ·

1 small sweet potato

2 tablespoons almond butter

Sprinkle of cinnamon

Sprinkle of flaxseeds

Preheat the oven to 375°F. Rinse the potato and pat it dry. Cut a piece of aluminum foil and place the sweet potato in the center. Poke the sweet potato with a fork on all sides, which will allow it to release steam and cook evenly. Loosely wrap the sweet potato in the foil, seal well, and place on a baking sheet. Bake 35 to 50 minutes or until it is soft and a knife can easily slide through the center. Remove the sweet potato and cut in half lengthwise. Spread with almond butter and sprinkle with cinnamon and flaxseeds.

> ➤ *SPOTLIGHT ON SWEET POTATOES*
> Sweet potatoes are among nature's richest sources of beta-carotene (vitamin A), which promotes healthy immune function and cellular growth. Since vitamin A is a fat-soluble vitamin, it's smart to consume some amount of fat like coconut oil, almond butter, or avocado with your sweet potato to reap the full benefits of this powerhouse veggie. Additionally, sweet potatoes are rich in easily digestible fiber. As you continue to take a break from grains and allow your digestive system to rest and restore, sweet potatoes can satisfy your yearning for comforting, grainy goodness.

Surfer's Delight

· · · · · · · · · · · · · · ·

1 cup water (more or less, depending on saucepan size)

2 teaspoons white vinegar

1 teaspoon sea salt

2 eggs

2 cups baby greens or arugula

¼ cup black beans, rinsed and drained

2 tablespoons guacamole (page 142)

2 tablespoons salsa (page 142)

Cilantro, for garnish

Green onion, for garnish

Add approximately 1 inch of water to a saucepan, along with the white vinegar and sea salt. Bring the water to a medium simmer. Crack the eggs into two separate small bowls or ramekins, keeping the yolks intact. Using a spoon, stir the heated water in one direction until it's spinning around like a whirlpool. Drop the eggs into the center of the whirlpool, cover the pan, and turn off the heat. Wait 5 to 6 minutes. While the eggs cook, place the baby greens on a plate. Top with the black beans, guacamole, and salsa. Garnish with chopped cilantro and green onion.

When the eggs are done, gently remove them from the pan with a large spoon and place them on top.

Midday and Early-Evening Juices

Both juice recipes make 16 ounces.

Crimson Berry

· · · · · · · · · · · · · · ·

2 carrots

½ raw unpeeled beet

1 medium cucumber (with skin)

½ cup blueberries

1 lemon, peeled

½ inch unpeeled gingerroot

½ teaspoon ground turmeric

Juice all the ingredients.

JUICE BAR BLEND: Carrot, beet, cucumber, lemon, ginger.

BLENDER RECIPE: Replace the fresh carrots with 8 ounces of pre-pressed carrot juice or coconut water. (You can get this at any health food store or juice shop.) Squeeze the lemon by hand and peel and grate the ginger before blending with all ingredients until smooth.

Life Line

. . . .

2 medium carrots

1 Granny Smith apple

½ medium raw unpeeled beet

1 medium cucumber (with skin)

½ teaspoon ground turmeric

Juice all the ingredients.

JUICE BAR BLEND: Carrot, apple, beet, cucumber, ginger.

BLENDER RECIPE: Replace fresh carrots or apple with 8 ounces of pre-pressed carrot juice or apple juice and chop all ingredients before adding to blender.

> ➤ *SPOTLIGHT ON BEETS*
> The ruby-red beet is packed with good-for-you vitamins, minerals, and antioxidants and is also a wonderful cleansing aid. The red betalin pigment in beets is a class of antioxidants that supports the body's metabolism and elimination of waste. Beets are a great source of iron and are known for their powerful anti-inflammatory qualities.

Midday Meals

Roasted Ruby Salad

. . . .

3 medium-size beets

Baby greens (as much as desired)

½ avocado

2 tablespoons chopped walnuts

Balsamic vinegar, for drizzling

Sea salt, to taste

Preheat the oven to 400°F. Slice off the beet greens and use them as an additional green in any of the juices this week. Scrub the beets and wrap them loosely in foil (it's okay if they're still wet). Place the wrapped beets on a baking sheet and bake for approximately an hour, or until a knife can easily slide through. Remove the beets and allow them to cool. If they are sufficiently cooked, the beet skin should peel away easily when you rub it off under running water in a sink.

Prepare a bed of baby greens on a plate. Dice the avocado and beets and add to the greens. Sprinkle the chopped walnuts on top. Drizzle the plate with balsamic vinegar and sprinkle with sea salt. This salad is so flavorful from the beets, creamy from the avocado, and crunchy from the walnuts that balsamic vinegar is really all you need to bring out the sweet delicious flavor—although if you'd like to dress your beets up a little bit more, give them a kiss of lemon (recipe below).

Lemon-Kissed Salad Dressing

- 1/2 cup purified water
- Juice of 2 lemons
- Pinch of stevia powder
- 2 tablespoons low-sodium tamari
- 1 tablespoon Dijon mustard
- 2 teaspoons garlic powder
- 1 tablespoon finely chopped parsley
- 1/2 teaspoon onion powder
- 1/4 teaspoon cayenne (optional)

Stir the water and lemon juice together until well mixed. Add stevia until your desired sweetness is achieved, using a whisk to avoid clumps if you're using powdered stevia. Add the rest of the ingredients to the mix and whisk well. Store unused dressing in an airtight container for up to 5 days.

San Diego Sando

- 2 butter lettuce leaves
- 4 ounces sliced turkey breast
- 1 tablespoon Dijon mustard
- 1/2 cup pea sprouts
- 1 medium tomato
- 1/2 avocado

Place two large, unbroken butter lettuce leaves on a plate. Using oven-roasted sliced turkey breast or nitrate-free low-sodium turkey meat, lay three or four slices on top of each leaf. Spread Dijon mustard over the turkey, then place sprouts on top. Slice the tomato and place two slices on top of the sprouts. Slice the avocado and put it on top of the tomato. Fold in half like a taco and enjoy!

Hot Bod Hummus Plate

· · · · · · · · · · · · · · · · · ·

3 cups torn romaine leaves

¼ avocado, cubed

¼ red onion, chopped

Sea salt, to taste

1 tablespoon balsamic vinegar

⅓ cup hummus (recipe follows)

1 cup cherry tomatoes

Place the romaine, cubed avocado, chopped red onion, sea salt, and balsamic vinegar in a small mixing bowl. Gently massage the ingredients together with your hands, mashing the avocado into the greens to form a dressing with the balsamic. Transfer to a plate or bowl. Prepare the hummus and place a scoop right on top of the salad. Halve the cherry tomatoes and toss them on top as a garnish.

HUMMUS

1 can chickpeas, rinsed and drained, *or* 2 cups cooked fresh chickpeas

¼ cup freshly squeezed lemon juice

¼ cup tahini

1 teaspoon sea salt

½ teaspoon ground cumin

1 clove garlic, minced

1–2 tablespoons water (optional)

Place all the ingredients in a food processor. If you're using canned chickpeas, rinse and drain them before use. Process the mixture to a chunky or smooth consistency depending on your hummus texture preference.

Makes 3–4 servings

➤ *SPOTLIGHT ON CHICKPEAS AND TAHINI*
Chickpeas are fiber all-stars. Their fiber in combination with their impressive amount of plant-based protein helps regulate blood sugar and keep you satiated. Tahini, a paste made from sesame seeds, is another fantastic pantry staple because it's rich in calcium. It adds dairy-free creaminess to dressings and dips without adding cheese, milk, or cream.

Early-Evening Meals

Heavenly Halibut and Garlicky Greens

· · · · · · · · · · · · · · · · ·

1 (5-ounce) halibut fillet (or substitute rainbow trout)

1 teaspoon olive oil

1 clove garlic

Sea salt, to taste

Black pepper, to taste

½ lemon

2 cups spinach

Preheat the oven to 400°F and line a baking sheet with parchment paper. Place the halibut on the parchment paper and rub the top with olive oil. Finely chop the garlic, reserve half, and spread the remaining garlic over the halibut fillet. Sprinkle the fillet with sea salt and black pepper. Slice the lemon half and place whole slices on top of the fish, allowing the citrus to infuse its flavor while baking. Bake the halibut for 12 to 18 minutes, depending on how cooked you prefer your fish.

While the halibut bakes, place a steamer basket over a saucepan with water and bring to a boil. Place the spinach in the steamer basket and put the lid on. Allow it to steam for 4 to 6 minutes, until it's wilted. Place the spinach on a plate, alongside the halibut, and sprinkle the greens with salt, pepper, and the reserved garlic. Enjoy the garlicky goodness!

Kale-ifornia Salad 2.0

· · · · · · · · · · · · · · · · ·

1 head kale

½ red onion, diced

1 whole avocado, cubed

1½ tablespoons tamari

2 tablespoons Dijon mustard

1 tablespoon garlic powder

1 pint cherry tomatoes

½ cup roasted butternut squash

2 tablespoons pumpkin seeds

Wash the kale and remove the tough stem with a sharp knife by slicing lengthwise down the center on each side of it. Stack the kale leaves on top of each other and finely chop into thin ribbons. Place the kale in a bowl. Add the red onion, avocado, tamari, Dijon, and garlic powder to the bowl. Using your hands, massage all of the ingredients together for 2 to 3 minutes, allowing the kale to soften and the avocado to form a creamy dressing with the tamari and Dijon. Halve the cherry tomatoes and cube the butternut squash. Gently toss them into the salad and garnish with pumpkin seeds.

Makes 2 servings

Liquid Sunshine

3 large carrots, chopped

1 teaspoon grated ginger

1½ teaspoons curry powder

½ teaspoon ground turmeric

1 stalk lemongrass, finely sliced

Sea salt, to taste

Chili flakes, to taste, plus more for garnish

1 onion, chopped

1½ cups vegetable broth (avoid added yeast and sugar)

1 can coconut milk

Grated carrot, for garnish

Cook the carrots, ginger, curry, turmeric, lemongrass, sea salt, chili flakes, and onion in the vegetable broth on the stovetop over medium heat for approximately half an hour, until the carrots are very tender. Transfer the mixture to a blender and puree until smooth. Pour the mixture back into the saucepan over medium heat. Add the coconut milk, stirring until creamy and smooth. Add grated carrot and chili flakes to garnish.

Makes 4 servings

> ➤ *SPOTLIGHT ON TURMERIC*
> Due to its anti-inflammatory and antioxidant properties, turmeric, a relative of ginger, has been shown in numerous studies to protect against a number of ailments. Its chief active compound, curcumin—which is what gives the spice its golden-yellow color—is thought to help protect and support liver function and boost immunity.

Week 2 Grab 'n' Go Snack Ideas

Choose one of these snacks if you get hungry late morning:

1 small Granny Smith apple, peach, pear, plum, or nectarine

1 (single-serving) packet raw almond or sunflower butter on celery sticks

10–15 raw walnuts or macadamia nuts

1 hard-boiled egg

4 ounces nitrate-free turkey slices

Week 2 Create-Your-Own Meals

This week, you're invited to create your own morning, midday, and early-evening meals by combining ingredients from the charts below. For either the Meat Eater's or Vegetarian options, choose one ingredient from each column.

Meat Eater's Meal

PROTEIN	FRESH GREEN VEGGIES	HEALTHY FATS
4 ounces lean protein	Unlimited	1 medium fresh fruit or ½ cup starchy veggies + 1 tablespoon healthy fat

Vegetarian Meal

PROTEIN	STARCHY VEGGIES	GREEN VEGGIES	HEALTHY FATS
¾ cup legumes	½ cup or 1 medium fresh fruit	Unlimited	1 tablespoon healthy oil, or 2 tablespoons nuts, or ⅓ avocado

WEEK 2 SHOPPING LIST

Your week 2 shopping list includes all the ingredients you'll need to create the rein-force juices and whole-food recipes. For a complete list of all the foods and ingredients that make the "In Crowd" this week, refer back to chapter 8, page 88. This week you're welcome to create your own nutritious and delicious dishes from the comprehensive list of week 2 "In Crowd" foods.

Fresh Produce

- Arugula
- Baby greens
- Beets
- Beet greens
- Butter lettuce
- Butternut squash
- Carrots
- Celery
- Cucumber
- Dandelion greens
- Green onion
- Kale
- Pea sprouts
- Red onion
- Romaine leaf lettuce
- Spinach
- Sweet potato

Fresh Whole Fruit

- Apples (Granny Smith only)
- Avocados
- Berries (blackberry, blueberry, raspberry, strawberry)
- Lemons
- Limes
- Nectarines
- Peaches
- Pears
- Pineapple (fresh in juices only)
- Plums
- Tomatoes (cherry, Roma)

Proteins

- Beans—black beans, chickpeas
- Eggs (organic, free-range)
- Lunch meat turkey and chicken (organic, low sodium, nitrate-free)
- Turkey (organic, oven-roasted)
- Wild-caught or sustainably farmed halibut, or rainbow trout

Healthy Fats: Nuts, Seeds, and Butters

(Preferably unroasted, unsalted, and unsweetened)

- Almonds and almond butter
- Chia seeds
- Flaxseeds
- Macadamia nuts
- Pumpkin seeds
- Tahini
- Walnuts

Fresh and Dried Herbs

This week prepare juices and whole-food meals with dried or fresh:

Cilantro	Mint
Ginger, gingerroot	Parsley (flat-leaf)

Spices and Seasonings

This week prepare juices and whole-food meals with dried or fresh:

Black pepper	Garlic, garlic powder
Cardamom	Lemongrass
Cayenne pepper	Nutmeg
Chili flakes	Onion powder
Cinnamon	Sea salt
Cumin	Serrano chile
Curry powder	Turmeric

Natural Sweeteners and Non-Dairy Milk

Almond milk (unsweetened)	Coconut water (unsweetened)
Coconut milk (unsweetened)	Stevia (organic or "whole leaf")

Essential Oils and Pantry Staples

Apple cider vinegar	Dijon mustard
Balsamic vinegar	Extra-virgin olive oil
Broth, vegetable and chicken (low sodium, no yeast or sugar)	Ghee (clarified butter)
	Tamari
	White vinegar

Week 3 Recipes at a Glance

JUICES
Arise

Melon Spice

Wholesome Harvest

Grounded

MORNING MEALS
Peaches and Cream

Sunrise Apple Pie

Awaken to Bacon

MIDDAY MEALS
Turned-Up Tabbouleh

Berry Nutty Salad

No-Flaw Slaw

EARLY-EVENING MEALS
Amazin' Asian Sea Bass

Mexicali Mixer

Tangy 'n' Tropical Black Beans

DESSERTS
Coconutty Lemon Burst Truffles

Brownies Done Better

CHAPTER 14

WEEK 3: RECHARGE
Recipes + shopping guide

Morning Juice Hydration

Both juice recipes make 16 ounces.

Arise

. . . .

4 oranges, peeled

1/4 whole pineapple, peeled and cored

1/2 cup basil

Pinch of cardamom powder

Pinch of cayenne powder

4-6 ounces water

Juice the oranges, pineapple, and basil, then stir in the cardamom and cayenne.

JUICE BAR BLEND: Orange, pineapple, lemon.

BLENDER RECIPE: Replace the fresh oranges with 8 ounces pre-pressed orange juice or 8 ounces coconut water. Blend until smooth.

Melon Spice

. . . .

1/2 small cantaloupe (rind and seeds removed)

1 lemon, peeled

1 inch unpeeled gingerroot

1-3 ounces water

Pinch of cayenne pepper

Stevia, to taste (optional)

Juice the cantaloupe, lemon, and ginger. Mix in the water and cayenne and stir in the stevia if desired.

JUICE BAR BLEND: Cantaloupe, lemon, ginger.

BLENDER RECIPE: Squeeze the lemon by hand and peel the ginger before blending all the ingredients until smooth.

➤ *SPOTLIGHT ON CAYENNE*
Cayenne pepper is much more than a flavorful and fiery spice. Studies have shown that cayenne may help to decrease appetite and burn calories. In addition to capsaicin, which gives cayenne its heat, the pepper contains nutrients including vitamins A and C, as well as carotenoids that have healthful antioxidant properties.

Morning Meals
Peaches and Cream

. . . .

NOTE: This is a make-the-night-before recipe. Planning ahead is necessary.

- 1 cup unsweetened goat's or sheep's yogurt
- 1 tablespoon chia seeds
- 2 tablespoons oat bran
- 1 tablespoon ground flaxseeds
- 1 teaspoon cinnamon
- 1 peach
- Dash of maple syrup (optional)

The night before, add the yogurt, chia seeds, oats, flax, and cinnamon to a bowl or mason jar. Mix together well and place in the fridge. In the morning, slice half of a peach to top and drizzle with a bit of maple syrup to taste. Alternatively, you can slice a whole peach to top and skip the maple syrup.

VARIATION: If you're avoiding dairy, feel free to use a non-dairy milk to make a chia pudding as in previous weeks. Follow the base chia seed pudding recipe mixing in 2 tablespoons oats and 1 tablespoon flaxseeds; use cinnamon, peaches, and maple syrup as the toppings.

Sunrise Apple Pie

. . . .

- 1 small raw Fuji apple
- 2 tablespoons almond or sunflower butter
- 1 teaspoon cinnamon
- ½ teaspoon nutmeg
- 1 teaspoon flaxseeds
- 1 tablespoon water

Preheat the oven to 375°F. Using an apple corer or melon baller, core the apple to approximately ½ inch of the bottom so the end is still closed. In a small bowl, mix together the almond or sunflower butter, cinnamon, nutmeg, and flaxseeds. Fill the core with this mixture and place the apple in a small baking dish, oven-safe bowl, or custard dish. Add about a tablespoon of water to the dish and bake for 30 to 35 minutes until tender.

> ➤ *SPOTLIGHT ON FLAXSEEDS*
> Flaxseeds contain heart-healthy omega-3 fatty acids, which are also beneficial to the skin. They are rich in lignans—phytochemicals that help balance hormones. They are also very high in both soluble and insoluble fiber, which helps stabilize blood sugar and regulate digestion.

Awaken to Bacon

. . . .

2 slices nitrate-free turkey bacon

1 cup water (more or less, depending on size of saucepan)

2 teaspoons white vinegar

1 teaspoon sea salt plus finishing sprinkle, to taste

2 eggs

2 cups arugula

¼ avocado

1 tomato, sliced

Cracked pepper, to taste

Line a baking sheet with foil and arrange the bacon slices on the sheet. Place the baking sheet in a cold oven and turn the heat on to 400°F. Bake 15 to 20 minutes, until golden brown. In the meantime, add approximately 1 inch of water to a saucepan along with the white vinegar and 1 teaspoon of the sea salt. Bring the water to a medium simmer. Crack the eggs into two separate small bowls or ramekins, keeping the yolks intact. Using a spoon, stir the heated water in one direction until it's spinning around like a whirlpool. Drop the eggs into the center of the whirlpool, cover the pan, and turn off the heat. Wait 5 to 6 minutes. Arrange the arugula on a plate, and add the poached eggs on top. Slice the avocado and tomato and place next to the eggs. Sprinkle with sea salt and freshly cracked black pepper. Remove the bacon from the oven and break over the eggs.

Midday and Early-Evening Juices

Wholesome Harvest

. . . .

2 medium carrots

1 Fuji apple

1 orange, peeled

½ medium cucumber (with skin)

1 lime, peeled

3 sprigs cilantro or flat-leaf parsley

¼ teaspoon ground turmeric

Juice all the ingredients.

JUICE BAR BLEND: Carrot, apple, orange, cucumber, lime.

BLENDER RECIPE: Replace the fresh carrots and apples with 8 ounces of pre-pressed carrot or apple juice, or 8 ounces coconut water. Juice the lime by hand. Blend all the ingredients until smooth.

Grounded

· · · · · · · · · · · · · ·

2 carrots

2 stalks celery

1 cup spinach

1 cucumber (with skin)

½ cup beet greens

Juice all the ingredients.

JUICE BAR BLEND: Carrot, celery, spinach, cucumber.

BLENDER RECIPE: Replace the fresh carrots and celery with 8 ounces unsweetened coconut water or pre-pressed carrot juice from a juice bar or grocery juice counter. Blend all the ingredients until smooth.

> ➤ *SPOTLIGHT ON CARROTS*
> They don't call them "the crunchy power food" for nothing; carrots provide tons of nutrition to the body, and did we mention they're delicious? Carrots are the second most popular vegetable in the world, after potatoes. If you know anything about carrot nutrition, you know they're chock-full of beta-carotene. Believe it or not, the nutrient beta-carotene was named after the carrot! They're an incredible source of vitamin A; immune-supportive vitamin C; bone-building vitamin K; and heart-healthy dietary fiber and potassium.

Midday Meals

Turned-Up Tabbouleh

· · · · · · · · · · · · · ·

1 cup quinoa

2 cups low-sodium vegetable broth

1 tablespoon chopped parsley

1 small cucumber

½ small red onion

½ pint cherry tomatoes

1 ounce soft goat's cheese

½ lemon

1 teaspoon olive oil

1 teaspoon garlic powder

Sea salt, to taste

3 ounces baked or grilled chicken breast, sliced

Put the quinoa and low-sodium vegetable broth in a medium saucepan, bring to a boil, then reduce heat to low. Cover the quinoa and allow to cook for 15 minutes. Remove the pot from the stove and let it sit, covered, for 5 minutes. Remove the lid and fluff with a fork. Add ½ cup of the quinoa to a mixing bowl and save the rest for another meal. Add the parsley, cucumber, red onion, and cherry tomatoes. Crumble in some goat's cheese. Squeeze the juice of ½ lemon into the bowl and add the olive oil, garlic powder, and sea salt to taste. Mix well and transfer to a serving bowl. Slice chicken and place on top.

Berry Nutty Salad

. . . .

3 cups mixed baby greens

2 ounces crumbled soft goat's cheese

1 tablespoon chopped walnuts

½ cup strawberries, quartered

1½ tablespoons balsamic vinegar

Sea salt, to taste

Pepper, to taste

Add the baby greens, goat's cheese, chopped walnuts, strawberries, balsamic vinegar, sea salt, and pepper to a bowl and toss together well until the ingredients are evenly distributed. Transfer to a serving bowl and enjoy.

No-Flaw Slaw

. . . .

¾ red cabbage, shredded or thinly sliced

¾ cup white cabbage, shredded or thinly sliced

⅓ cup grated carrot

4 green onions, chopped

¼ cup chopped flat-leaf parsley

3 ounces roasted skinless chicken breast, diced

2 tablespoons sunflower seeds

1 small lemon, juiced

2 teaspoons flax oil

1 clove garlic, minced

1 tablespoon tamari

Add all the ingredients to a bowl and mix well until the veggies are evenly distributed and thoroughly dressed (no need to make the dressing separately). This salad gets better over time, so making a larger batch for fridge leftovers or making it a day or two before you plan to eat it is a great idea.

Early-Evening Meals

Amazin' Asian Sea Bass

• • • • • • • • • • • • • •

5 ounces sea bass (or substitute striped bass)

1 tablespoon miso paste

1 tablespoon tamari

1 teaspoon grated ginger

Juice of ½ lemon

2 teaspoons garlic powder

1 cup asparagus

Sea salt, to taste

Black pepper

Sliced green onion, for garnish

Preheat the oven to 400°F and line a baking sheet with parchment paper. Place the sea bass on the parchment paper. Add the miso, tamari, ginger, lemon juice, and garlic powder to a blender and blend until smooth. Pour over the sea bass and rub into the fish so it is thoroughly marinated. Bake the sea bass for 12 to 18 minutes, depending on how cooked you prefer your fish. While the fish bakes, place a steamer basket over a saucepan with water and bring to a boil. Place the asparagus in the steamer basket and put the lid on, allowing it to steam for 4 to 6 minutes, or until tender. Place the asparagus on a plate alongside the fish and sprinkle with sea salt and black pepper. Add green onion to garnish.

Mexicali Mixer

. . . .

3 ounces sliced beef or bison steak

3 cups romaine lettuce

½ cup cooked black, kidney, or pinto beans, canned or fresh

1 batch avocado salsa (see below)

1 green onion, for garnish

AVOCADO SALSA

2 vine-ripened or Roma tomatoes

½ small onion

1 clove garlic, minced

2 tablespoons cilantro, chopped

Sea salt, to taste

¼ teaspoon cayenne, or to taste if you prefer spicier

Juice of ½ lemon

Juice of 1 small lime

¼ avocado, diced

Bake or grill the meat to your preference and allow to rest and cool. Arrange the romaine in a bowl. Drain and rinse a can of black beans or use fresh cooked on the stovetop. Add the beans to the romaine. To make the avocado salsa, add the tomatoes, onion, garlic, cilantro, sea salt, cayenne, lemon juice, and lime juice to the food processor. Process until the salsa is mixed together but still chunky. Pour into a small bowl and stir in the diced avocado. Pour over the black beans and add the sliced steak on top. Chop the green onion and sprinkle over to garnish.

Tangy 'n' Tropical Black Beans

. . . .

1 cup cooked black beans, canned or fresh

¼ medium mango, diced

½ cup diced jicama

½ red bell pepper, diced

¼ medium red onion, diced

¼ avocado, diced

1 tablespoon chopped cilantro

2 teaspoons garlic powder

Juice of 1 small lime

Sea salt, to taste

Cayenne pepper, to taste

Use fresh black beans cooked over the stovetop or drain and rinse 1 cup of low-sodium canned black beans. Add them to a bowl along with the mango, jicama, bell pepper, red onion, avocado, cilantro, garlic powder, and lime juice. Mix well and sprinkle with sea salt and cayenne to taste.

Desserts

Coconutty Lemon Burst Truffles

· · · · · · · · · · · · · · · · · ·

½ cup almonds

½ cup unsweetened shredded coconut

Pinch of sea salt

3 tablespoons coconut oil

2 tablespoons lemon zest

Process the almonds in the food processor until a fine meal is formed. Add it to a bowl with the remaining ingredients and mix well until it becomes a dough that holds together. Roll into small truffles and place on a flat plate or parchment-lined cutting board. Keep in the refrigerator, allowing them to slightly harden. The truffles will remain fresh for approximately 1 week.

Makes 10–12 truffles; serving size is 1 or 2

VARIATION: You can substitute orange zest or cinnamon for the lemon zest.

> ➤ *SPOTLIGHT ON COCONUT*
> All around, coconut is rich in fiber, vitamins, and minerals. Coconut meat (the dried and shredded stuff in a bag) is relatively low in carbohydrates and high in fiber. Coconut oil is composed of medium-chain fatty acids (MCFAs) and is high in lauric acid, a type of saturated fat that may actually help to raise healthy HDL cholesterol levels and maintain healthy gut bacteria. Sweet and satisfying coconut milk may help keep overall body fat, as well as your waistline, in check. When the MCFAs in coconut are consumed, they go directly from the intestines to the liver to be burned as fuel, rather than being stored as body fat.

Brownies Done Better

· · · · · · · · · · · · · · · · · ·

1 cup almond butter

½ cup maple syrup

2 tablespoons coconut oil

1 egg

1 teaspoon vanilla extract

⅓ cup cacao powder

½ teaspoon baking soda

1 tablespoon decaf espresso powder

½ teaspoon coarse sea salt, plus more to sprinkle on top if desired

Preheat the oven to 325°F. In a large bowl, mix together the almond butter, maple syrup, coconut oil, egg, and vanilla. When the liquid is well mixed, stir in the cacao powder, baking soda, espresso powder, and sea salt. Pour the batter into a parchment-lined or coconut-oiled 9 x 9-inch baking pan. Sprinkle a pinch of sea salt over the top of the brownies if desired. Bake for 20 to 25 minutes, until the brownies have formed a nice flaky skin but are still chewy and soft in the middle.

Makes 9 brownies; serving size is 1

Did You Know?

Espresso and chocolate are a match made in heaven! The espresso in Brownies Done Better is almost undetectable but really brings out the chocolaty flavor. Meanwhile the sea salt highlights the sweetness of the maple syrup.

Week 3 Grab 'n' Go Snack Ideas

Choose one of the following if you get hungry late morning:

1 medium banana

1 tablespoon almond or sunflower butter on a brown rice cake

1 hard-boiled egg

1 cup unsweetened goat's or sheep's yogurt with 1/2 cup berries

Week 3 Create-Your-Own Meals

This week, you're invited to create your own morning, midday, and early-evening meals by combining ingredients from the charts below. For each option, choose one ingredient from each column.

Meat Eater's Meal

PROTEIN	FRESH GREEN VEGGIES	STARCH	FAT
5 ounces animal protein (from in-crowd options)	Unlimited	1/2 cup starchy veggies, legumes, or gluten-free grains	1 tablespoon healthy fat, or 2 tablespoons nuts, or 1/3 avocado

Vegetarian Meal

PROTEIN	FRESH GREEN VEGGIES	STARCH	FAT
3/4 cup legumes	Unlimited	1/2 cup starchy veggies or gluten-free grains	1 tablespoon healthy fat, or 2 tablespoons nuts, or 1/3 avocado

WEEK 3 SHOPPING LIST

Your week 3 shopping list includes all the ingredients you'll need to create the recharge juices and whole-food recipes. For a complete list of all the foods and ingredients that make the "In Crowd" this week, refer back to chapter 9, page 105. Throughout the week, you're welcome to create your own nutritious and delicious dishes from the comprehensive list of week 3 "In Crowd" foods.

Fresh Produce

Arugula

Asparagus

Baby greens

Beet greens

Cabbage

Carrots

Celery

Cucumber

Green onion

Jicama

Red bell pepper

Red onion

Romaine leaf lettuce

Spinach

Fresh Whole Fruit

Apples (Fuji)

Avocados

Bananas

Cantaloupe (in juices only)

Kiwi

Lemons

Limes

Mango

Oranges

Peaches

Pineapple

Strawberries

Tomatoes (cherry, Roma)

Gluten-Free Grains

Brown rice cakes (low sodium and sugar free)

Oat bran

Quinoa

Proteins

Beans—black, kidney, pinto

Beef (grass-fed)

Bison (grass-fed)

Chicken (organic, skinless, white meat)

Eggs (organic, free-range)

Turkey (organic, oven-roasted), and turkey bacon (nitrate-free)

Wild-caught or sustainably farmed sea bass or striped bass

Dairy

Goat's cheese, yogurt (unsweetened)

Sheep's yogurt (unsweetened)

Healthy Fats: Nuts, Seeds, and Butters

(Preferably unroasted, unsalted, and unsweetened)

- Almonds and almond butter
- Chia seeds
- Flaxseeds
- Sunflower seeds and sunflower butter
- Walnuts

Fresh and Dried Herbs

This week prepare juices and whole-food meals with dried or fresh:

- Basil
- Cilantro
- Ginger, gingerroot
- Parsley (flat-leaf)

Spices and Seasonings

This week prepare juices and whole-food meals with dried or fresh:

- Black pepper
- Cardamom
- Cayenne pepper
- Cinnamon
- Cracked pepper
- Garlic, garlic powder
- Nutmeg
- Sea salt
- Turmeric

Natural Sweeteners

- Almond milk (unsweetened)
- Cacao powder
- Coconut milk (unsweetened)
- Coconut water (unsweetened)
- Maple syrup
- Shredded coconut (unsweetened)
- Stevia (organic or "whole leaf")
- Vanilla extract

Essential Oils and Pantry Staples

- Baking soda
- Balsamic vinegar
- Broth, vegetable and chicken (low sodium, no yeast or sugar)
- Coconut oil
- Cold-pressed flax oil
- Decaf espresso powder
- Extra-virgin olive oil
- Ghee (clarified butter)
- Miso
- Tamari
- White vinegar

Week 4 Recipes at a Glance

JUICES
Mediterranean

Watermelon Breeze

The Greens

Island Greens

MORNING MEALS
Banana Cream Chia Oatmeal

Sunny Side Sammy

Better Bacon Omelet

MIDDAY MEALS
Bliss Burgers

Mediterranean Medley

Never-Fail Kale Salad

EARLY-EVENING MEALS
Beach Bum Burritacos

Seared Scallops in the Sand

Oh My Thai Bowl

DESSERTS
Sunflower Power Cookies

Cacao Almond Super Snacks

CHAPTER 15
· · · · · · · · ·
WEEK 4: RENEW
Recipes + shopping guide

Morning Juice Hydration

Both juice recipes make 12 ounces.

Mediterranean

· · · · · · · · · · · · · · · ·

½ fennel bulb

2 lemons, peeled

3 oranges, peeled

1 sprig mint

3-4 ounces water

1 teaspoon apple cider vinegar

Stevia, to taste (optional)

Juice the fennel, lemons, oranges, mint, and water. Stir in apple cider vinegar and stevia if needed.

JUICE BAR BLEND: Celery, cucumber, lemon, orange.

BLENDER RECIPE: Peel the lemon and the oranges before blending all the ingredients until smooth.

➤ *SPOTLIGHT ON APPLE CIDER VINEGAR AND MINT*

Both apple cider vinegar and mint infuse flavor into your morning juices and pack a nutritional punch. Apple cider vinegar also contains acetic acid, which may lessen your appetite and speed up metabolism. Fresh mint (spearmint and peppermint) is a potent antioxidant and contains trace amounts of iron, vitamin A, and potassium.

Watermelon Breeze

· · · · · · · · · · · · · · · ·

½ small watermelon (remove rind)

4 sprigs mint

½ fennel bulb

1 lime, peeled

Stevia, to taste (optional)

Remove the watermelon skin by cutting lengthwise from top to bottom along the flesh and the rind. Juice the watermelon, mint, fennel, and lime. Stir in stevia if needed.

JUICE BAR BLEND: Watermelon, lime.

BLENDER RECIPE: Add 4 ounces coconut water. Squeeze the lime by hand and blend all the ingredients until smooth.

Morning Meals
Banana Cream Chia Oatmeal

. . . .

½ cup dry oats

¼ cup unsweetened milk of your choice (cow's, goat's, sheep's, coconut, almond)

¼ cup water

1 tablespoon chia seeds

1 teaspoon cinnamon

½ teaspoon nutmeg

½ teaspoon cardamom

Pinch of sea salt

½ ripe banana

1 tablespoon walnuts, chopped

Sprinkle of shredded coconut

Stevia, to taste (optional)

Combine the oats, milk, water, chia seeds, cinnamon, nutmeg, cardamom, and sea salt in a saucepan over medium heat. Slice the banana into the pan; allow the oatmeal to heat to a soft bubbly steam, stirring. Continue to stir well to allow the banana to break down into the oats. Do this for 5 to 7 minutes until the oats have absorbed the liquid. Pour into a bowl and top with chopped walnuts and shredded coconut. Add stevia as desired.

Sunny Side Sammy

. . . .

1 tablespoon coconut oil or ghee

2 eggs

2 slices sprouted wheat bread

½ avocado

2–3 slices tomato

Sea salt, to taste

Cracked pepper, to taste

Chili flakes, to taste (optional)

Place a skillet over medium heat and add the coconut oil or ghee. Allow the pan to heat up, then crack two eggs directly into it. Let them cook until the whites have turned opaque. Cover the pan and lower the heat, allowing the steam to cook the tops of the eggs. In the meantime, toast two slices of sprouted wheat bread. Slice the avocado and tomato and place on the toast. Remove the lid from the eggs after 3 to 4 minutes, or when the yolks are cooked to your desired hardness. Place the eggs on top of the avocado-tomato toast and sprinkle with sea salt, cracked pepper, and, if desired, chili flakes to taste. The bread is a great "mop" for the runny yolk.

Better Bacon Omelet

2 slices bacon of your choice (turkey or pork, preferably nitrate-free)

2 eggs

Sea salt, to taste

Black pepper, to taste

1½ teaspoons coconut oil or ghee

1 cup spinach (or any green leafy veggie)

1 medium tomato

Line a baking sheet with foil and arrange the bacon slices on the sheet. Place in an oven (do not preheat) and turn the heat to 400°F. Bake 15 to 20 minutes, until golden brown. In the meantime, whisk together the eggs, sea salt, and black pepper in a small bowl. Set the mixture aside. Place a skillet over medium heat and add the coconut oil or ghee, allowing it to heat up. While this happens, roughly chop the spinach into smaller pieces and slice the tomato. When the oil or ghee is heated, pour the egg mixture into the skillet and allow it to cook for a minute or two until the bottom is golden brown. Add the spinach and tomato to one side of the omelet. With a spatula, flip the other side over the filling and turn the heat to low, letting the whole omelet cook for another minute or two. Transfer to a plate alongside the bacon, and enjoy.

Midday and Early-Evening Juices

Both juice recipes make 8 ounces.

The Greens

· · · · · · · · · · · · · · · · ·

5 green apples

3 green kale leaves

3 green chard leaves

½ head green leaf lettuce

1 green bell pepper (seeds removed)

Juice all the ingredients.

JUICE BAR BLEND: Apple, kale, romaine, celery.

BLENDER RECIPE: Replace the fresh apples with 8 ounces of pre-pressed apple juice. You can find this at your local health food store or juice shop. Blend all the ingredients until smooth.

Island Greens

· · · · · · · · · · · · · · · · ·

3 medium cucumbers (with skin)

2 Granny Smith apples

1 cup spinach

4 collard leaves

1–2 kale leaves

5 sprigs mint

2 sprigs cilantro

½ inch lemongrass

4 limes, peeled

Juice all the ingredients.

JUICE BAR BLEND: Apple, cucumber, spinach, kale, lemon, lime.

BLENDER RECIPE: Replace the fresh apples with 8 ounces of pre-pressed apple juice. Replace the lemongrass with 1 lemon and squeeze both the lemon and limes by hand. Remove the cucumber skin and chop all veggies and herbs before blending until smooth.

> ➤ *SPOTLIGHT ON LIME*
> Limes are an excellent source of vitamins C and B₆, potassium, folate, and the phytochemical limonene, which helps to stimulate digestion. Lime also adds great flavor to food, juices, and tonics without adding calories or fat.

Midday Meals

Bliss Burgers

. . . .

1 cup sunflower seeds

½ cup brown rice or whole rolled oats, cooked

1 cup water

½ cup shredded carrots

2 cloves garlic

2 teaspoons onion powder

2 tablespoons chopped flat-leaf parsley

2 tablespoons chopped chives

1 teaspoon sea salt

Preheat the oven to 400°F. Pulse the sunflower seeds in a food processor until they are broken up into smaller pieces, but still chunky—they give great texture. Add the rest of the ingredients and pulse until the mixture begins to hold together. If you prefer a less chunky consistency to your burger, you can process the mixture until it forms a dough. Take a scoop of the mixture and form into a patty shape, repeating this until you have approximately six patties. Place them on a parchment-lined baking sheet and bake at 400°F for 20 minutes. You want to set a timer for 10 minutes and flip them midway through. These may be kept in the fridge or frozen for future meals.

Makes 6 burgers; serving size is 1

TIP: If you're using whole rolled oats, add more water to the mixture if it seems dry. Oats tend to be drier than cooked brown rice.

➤ *SPOTLIGHT ON OATS*

There are so many oat products in the bulk grain and cereal section, it can be a little confusing when making your choices. The four common varieties are steel cut, whole rolled oats, quick oats, and instant oats. These are all made from an oat groat, which is the whole grain of oat before anything has been done to it. Steel-cut oats are simply the groat with the hull removed, and cut into several pieces with a steel blade. They have the least amount of processing and retain a nutty flavor and chewy texture. "Old-fashioned" or whole rolled oats are whole grains of oats that are steamed and flattened out between rollers. Since the steaming process partially cooks the oats, they cook faster on your stovetop than steel-cut oats. Quick oats are rolled oats that have been steamed even longer and rolled out even flatter to make them cook very quickly. They have less texture than thick rolled oats. Instant oats are rolled thinner still, into an almost powder-like substance. This is the variety often found in "instant oatmeal" packets. Not only are instant oats the least nutritious kind, but also they're very often loaded with salt and added sugars when purchased in the flavored packets.

Mediterranean Medley

· · · · · · · · · · · · · · ·

²/₃ cup chopped flat-leaf parsley

1 medium cucumber, diced

¹/₂ medium red onion, diced

1 pint cherry tomatoes, halved

1 cup cooked wheat berries, quinoa, or brown rice

Juice of ¹/₂ lemon

1 tablespoon olive oil

1 teaspoon garlic powder

1 tablespoon red wine vinegar

Sea salt, to taste

3 cups baby greens

Hummus (see below)

Sprinkle of paprika, for garnish

Combine the parsley, cucumber, red onion, and cherry tomatoes in a mixing bowl with 1 cup cooked grain of your choice. Squeeze the juice of half a lemon into the bowl and add the olive oil, garlic powder, red wine vinegar, and sea salt to taste. Mix well and place half of the chopped salad on top of a plated bed of baby greens. This salad keeps well because the flavors have more time to marinate together, so wrap the other half up for a future meal. Next, make the hummus in the food processor. Top the salad with ¹/₄ cup of hummus and garnish with a sprinkle of paprika.

HUMMUS

1 can chickpeas, rinsed and drained, *or* 2 cups cooked fresh chickpeas

¹/₄ cup freshly squeezed lemon juice

¹/₄ cup tahini

1 teaspoon sea salt

¹/₂ teaspoon ground cumin

1 clove garlic, minced

1–2 tablespoons water (optional)

Place all the ingredients in a food processor. If you're using canned chickpeas, rinse and drain them before use. Process the mixture to a chunky or smooth consistency depending on your hummus texture preference.

Makes 3–4 servings

Never-Fail Kale Salad

· · · · · · · · · · · · · · ·

1 head kale, de-stemmed

1/2 red onion, diced

1 whole avocado, cubed

1 1/2 tablespoons tamari

2 tablespoons Dijon mustard

1 tablespoon garlic powder

1 pint cherry tomatoes

1/2 cup cooked and cooled grain of your choice

2 tablespoons pine nuts

1 ounce soft goat's cheese

Wash the kale and finely chop using a good knife. Place the kale in a bowl. Add the red onion, avocado, tamari, Dijon, and garlic powder to the bowl. Using your hands, massage all of the ingredients together for 2 to 3 minutes, allowing the kale to soften and the avocado to form a creamy dressing with the other ingredients. Halve the cherry tomatoes and measure out the grain, pine nuts, and cheese. Gently toss them into the salad and enjoy.

Makes 2 servings

Early-Evening Meals

Beach Bum Burritacos

· · · · · · · · · · · · · · ·

1 cup beans of your choice, canned or fresh

2 handfuls arugula

2 mini sprouted whole wheat, brown rice, or corn tortillas

2 tablespoons guacamole (see below)

2 tablespoons salsa (see below)

1 ounce Cotija cheese crumbles

Green onion

GUACAMOLE

2 ripe avocados

2 tablespoons cilantro or flat-leaf parsley

1 clove garlic

2 tablespoons red onion

1 tablespoon lime juice

Sea salt, to taste

SALSA

3 whole vine-ripened or Roma tomatoes—if heirloom varieties are available to you, try these for a gorgeous rainbow of colors!

2 tablespoons chopped cilantro or flat-leaf parsley

1 small onion

4 green onions

1 seeded serrano chile (optional)

2 cloves garlic

Juice of 1 lime

Sea salt, to taste

Drain and rinse a can of black, kidney, or pinto beans, or use fresh cooked. Add a handful of arugula to the center of two mini tortillas and place ½ cup of the beans on top of each tortilla to keep the arugula in place.

Make the guacamole by roughly chopping the avocados, cilantro, garlic, and red onion and adding them to the food processor. Squeeze in the lime juice and sprinkle in sea salt to taste. Process the guacamole to your desired consistency and scoop on top of the beans.

Wash out the processor, then make the salsa by roughly chopping the tomatoes, cilantro, onion, green onions, serrano chile, and garlic and adding them to the food processor. Process until the salsa is mixed together but still chunky. Put a tablespoon of salsa on each tortilla. Sprinkle the Cotija cheese crumbles over the salsa. Finely chop the green onion and sprinkle to garnish.

Seared Scallops in the Sand

• • • • • • • • • • • • • • • • •

1 cup barley

3 cups low-sodium vegetable broth

1 teaspoon ghee or coconut oil

¼ medium onion, diced

½ clove garlic, minced

Juice of ½ large lemon

1 tablespoon chopped thyme

1 tablespoon chopped parsley

1 tablespoon chopped rosemary

1 medium tomato, diced

Sea salt, to taste

Black pepper, to taste

1 cup broccoli rabe

4 scallops

Put the barley and the low-sodium vegetable broth in a medium sauté pan, bring to a boil, and reduce the heat to low. Cover the barley and cook for 15 minutes. In the meantime, heat a skillet with the ghee or coconut oil and sauté the onion and garlic for a minute or two, watching to avoid burning the garlic. Add the lemon juice, herbs, tomato, sea salt, and black pepper. Let the mixture simmer for 4 to 5 minutes. While that cooks, place the broccoli rabe in a steamer basket and put the lid on. Allow it to steam for 5 to 7 minutes, until it is soft and the stems become pliable. While that steams, add the scallops to the simmering mixture in the sauté pan and cover. Cook for 2 minutes, until they are heated through and opaque without becoming tough and rubbery. Place the broccoli on the center of a plate and sprinkle with sea salt, black pepper, and a squeeze of lemon juice. Spoon ¾ cup of cooked barley into 4 small scoops around the broccoli, pressing down the center with the spoon to make a "bed" for the scallops, saving the rest of the barley in the fridge for a future meal. Place a scallop on top of each barley "bed" and pour the remaining sauté pan mixture over the scallops. Garnish with more chopped herbs.

Oh My Thai Bowl

1 cup brown rice

2½ cups low-sodium vegetable broth

1 cup broccoli

1 cup baby bok choy

1 tablespoon coconut oil

Sea salt, to taste

1 teaspoon ground ginger

1 tablespoon miso paste

2 tablespoons tamari

1 tablespoon garlic powder

1 tablespoon lemon juice

1 (4-ounce) salmon fillet

¼ avocado

Sesame seeds

Cook the brown rice in the low-sodium vegetable broth by bringing the rice and broth to a boil. Reduce the heat to low and simmer for 40 to 50 minutes with the lid on until most of the liquid has been absorbed. Let it stand for 5 minutes and remove to a bowl, fluffing with a fork. While the rice cooks, preheat the oven to 400°F and line a baking sheet with parchment paper. Toss the broccoli and whole baby bok choy in the coconut oil, sea salt, and ginger. Place on one half of the baking sheet. Add the miso, tamari, garlic powder, and lemon juice to a blender and blend until smooth. Pour over the salmon, rubbing the mixture in so the fish is well coated. Add the fish to the other side of the baking sheet; bake everything for 13 to 18 minutes, until the fish is cooked and the veggies are fork-tender. If the veggies take longer, pull the fish out when it's cooked to your desired doneness. Dice the avocado. Add ¾ cup of the cooked brown rice to a bowl and save the rest for a future meal. Add the roasted veggies, avocado, and salmon on top of the rice. Sprinkle the dish with sesame seeds and tamari to taste.

➤ *SPOTLIGHT ON SALMON*
Salmon is a superstar for its natural omega-3 fatty acids, which are believed to benefit the body in many ways, from mood to memory to heart health and beyond. It's also a wonderful source of protein that can be enjoyed smoked, baked, poached, seared, or grilled for variety.

Desserts

Sunflower Power Cookies

. . . .

1 cup sunflower butter

¾ cup coconut sugar

1 egg

Vanilla extract

¾ teaspoon baking soda

Coarse sea salt flakes, to sprinkle on top (optional)

Preheat the oven to 350°F and line a baking sheet with parchment paper. Mix the sunflower butter, coconut sugar, egg, vanilla extract, and baking soda until smooth and well combined. Drop the dough in even-size balls onto the baking sheet and press down with a fork in both directions to leave a criss-cross mark on the top of each cookie. Sprinkle with coarse sea salt and bake for 7 to 10 minutes until golden brown and chewy.

VARIATION: Try adding dark chocolate chips to this recipe for Sunflower Chocolate Chunk Cookies.

Makes 8–10 cookies; serving size is 1.

Cacao Almond Super Snacks

· · · · · · · · · · · · · ·

1 cup almonds

6 large dates

¼ cup almond butter

2 tablespoons cacao powder

1 tablespoon coconut oil

1 cup shredded coconut

Place all the ingredients except the coconut in a blender and mix until smooth. Using your hands, roll the mixture into small balls. Place the shredded coconut on a plate and roll the balls in the coconut, helping it stick by pressing it gently into them. Place the balls on a plate in the refrigerator until firm.

Makes 8–10 snacks; serving size is 1–2.

> ➤ *SPOTLIGHT ON CACAO*
> We love cacao (the darkest of the dark chocolate) and it loves us back! In an Australian study published in the *British Medical Journal*, researchers found dark chocolate consumption could improve heart health. It's also a rich source of magnesium, iron, dietary fiber, and antioxidants. Cacao is a healthy alternative to the conventional sugar-based "cocoa" used for baking, hot chocolate, desserts, and smoothies.

Week 4 Grab 'n' Go Snack Ideas

Vegan Options (choose one)

½ melon

Kale chips (all natural, sugar-free)

Mixed veggies of your choice + ¼ cup homemade hummus

Non-Vegan Options (choose one)

2 ounces nitrate-free beef jerky

1 hard-boiled egg + 1 piece of fresh fruit

1 mini sprouted whole wheat, brown rice, or corn tortilla with 1 ounce goat's cheddar

Week 4 Create-Your-Own Meals

This week, you're invited to create your own morning, midday, and early-evening meals by combining ingredients from the tables below.

Meat Eater's Meal

PROTEIN	FRESH GREEN VEGGIES	STARCH	FAT
5 ounces animal protein (from in-crowd options)	Unlimited	¾ cup starchy veggies, legumes, or gluten-free grains	1 tablespoon healthy fat, or 2 tablespoons nuts, or ⅓ avocado

Vegetarian Meal

FRESH GREEN VEGGIES	STARCH	FAT
Unlimited	¾ cup starchy veggies ¾ cup legumes ¾ cup gluten-free grains	1 tablespoon healthy fat, or 2 tablespoons nuts, or ⅓ avocado

WEEK 4 SHOPPING LIST

Your week 4 shopping list includes all the ingredients you'll need to create the renew juices and whole-food recipes. For a complete list of all the foods and ingredients that make the "In Crowd" this week, refer back to chapter 10, page 114. Throughout the week, you're welcome to create your own nutritious and delicious dishes from the comprehensive list of week 4 "In Crowd" foods.

Fresh Produce

Arugula	Green bell pepper
Baby greens	Green leaf lettuce
Bok choy	Green onion
Broccoli	Kale
Carrots	Leeks
Collard greens	Red onion
Cucumber	Spinach
Fennel	Swiss chard

Fresh Whole Fruit

Apples (all)

Avocados

Bananas

Dates

Lemons

Limes

Oranges

Tomatoes (any, cherry)

Watermelon

Grains

Barley

Brown rice

Corn tortillas

Oats (whole) and oat bran

Quinoa

Wheat (preferably sprouted) bread and tortillas

Wheat berries

Proteins

Bacon (pork or turkey, nitrate-free)

Beans— chickpeas, plus your choice of black beans, butter beans, cannellini beans, great northern beans, kidney beans, lentils, lima beans, navy beans, pinto beans

Beef jerky (nitrate-free, unsweetened)

Eggs (organic, free-range)

Wild-caught or sustainably farmed salmon and scallops

Dairy

Cow's milk, Cotija cheese (organic, unsweetened)

Goat's milk, cheese (organic, unsweetened)

Sheep's milk (organic, unsweetened)

Healthy Fats: Nuts, Seeds, and Butters

(Preferably unroasted, unsalted, and unsweetened)

Almonds and almond butter

Chia seeds

Flaxseeds

Pine nuts

Sesame seeds

Sunflower seeds and sunflower butter

Tahini

Walnuts

Fresh and Dried Herbs

This week prepare juices and whole-food meals with dried or fresh:

Chives

Cilantro

Fennel

Ginger, gingerroot

Mint

Parsley (flat-leaf)

Rosemary

Thyme

Spices and Seasonings

This week prepare juices and whole-food meals with dried or fresh:

Black pepper	Lemongrass
Cardamom	Nutmeg
Chili flakes	Onion powder
Cinnamon	Paprika
Cracked Pepper	Sea salt
Garlic, garlic powder	Serrano chile

Natural Sweeteners and Non-Dairy Milk

Almond milk (unsweetened)	Coconut water (unsweetened)
Cacao powder	Dark chocolate chips
Coconut milk (unsweetened)	Shredded coconut (unsweetened)
Coconut palm sugar	Stevia
	Vanilla extract

Essential Oils and Pantry Staples

Apple cider vinegar	Dijon mustard
Baking soda	Extra-virgin olive oil
Balsamic vinegar	Ghee (clarified butter)
Broth, vegetable and chicken (low sodium, no yeast or sugar)	Miso
	Red wine vinegar
Coconut oil	Tamari

Afternoon Tea Lattes

Minty Green Tea

12-14 ounces almond milk

¼ avocado

1–2 teaspoons matcha green tea

4 sprigs mint (remove stem)

Honey, to taste

Combine all the ingredients and blend until smooth.

Spiced Latte

2 ounces cold brew coffee (see tip below)

2 young coconuts, liquid (5-7 ounces) and meat (¼ cup), or use 6 ounces of canned coconut milk or cream, *plus* 4 ounces of coconut water

⅛ cup cacao powder

1 teaspoon black sesame paste

½ teaspoon cinnamon

Pinch of allspice

Pinch of nutmeg

¼ teaspoon vanilla extract

Coconut palm sugar, to taste

CHAPTER 16

BONUS HYDRATION

Combine all the ingredients (except the coconut palm sugar) and blend until smooth. Sweeten to taste.

Tip: To prepare cold brew concentrate, combine 1 cup ground coffee with 8 ounces water and allow to steep overnight in fridge.

Mexican Chocolate

1/4 cup young coconut meat (or 2 ounces canned coconut milk or cream)

8–10 ounces almond milk

1/4 cup cacao powder

1 teaspoon chia seeds

1 teaspoon ground flaxseeds

1/2 teaspoon cinnamon

1/2 orange, peeled

Pinch of orange zest

1/4 teaspoon vanilla extract

Pinch of ground habanero chile

Zest and juice of 1/2 medium orange

Honey, to taste

Combine all the ingredients (except the honey) and blend until smooth. Sweeten to taste.

Pre-Workout Juices

Orange Rush

2 medium carrots

2 oranges, peeled

1 apple

4 ounces coconut water

1/4 teaspoon ground turmeric

1 tablespoon chia seeds

Juice the carrots, oranges, apples, coconut water, and turmeric. Stir in the chia seeds. Allow 2 to 3 minutes for chia seeds to hydrate, stirring to avoid clumping.

Green Power

8 ounces almond milk

1 cup spinach

1/2 avocado

3 oranges, peeled

1/4 fennel bulb

1 tablespoon chia seeds

1/2 inch unpeeled gingerroot

Combine all the ingredients and blend until smooth.

Post-Workout Juices

Body Ease

· · · · · · · · · · · · · ·

2 medium carrots

2 Granny Smith apples

1/4 raw beet

1/4 inch unpeeled gingerroot

1/4 teaspoon ground turmeric

1 banana

Juice all the ingredients except the banana. Combine the juice with the banana and blend until smooth.

JUICE BAR BLEND: Carrot, apple, beet, banana, ginger.

BLENDER RECIPE: Replace the carrots with 8 ounces coconut water or carrot juice from your local health food store or juice shop. Chop the apples and beet into small pieces. Peel and grate the ginger and blend all the ingredients until smooth.

Green Boost

· · · · · · · · · · · · · ·

1/2 small watermelon, (remove rind)

1 medium cucumber (with skin)

1 cup spinach

2 collard leaves

2 lemons, peeled

1/4 teaspoon chlorella

1/4 teaspoon spirulina

Juice the watermelon, cukes, spinach, collard leaves, and lemons. Stir in the chlorella and spirulina.

JUICE BAR BLEND: Watermelon, cucumber, spinach, lemon.

BLENDER RECIPE: Juice the lemon by hand and chop all ingredients before blending until smooth.

Hangover Helpers

Revive

. . . .

4 medium carrots

1 lime, peeled

1/4 cantaloupe (remove rind and seeds)

1/4 whole pineapple, peeled and cored

1/4 banana

1/8 cup fresh goji berries or 1/2 teaspoon goji berry powder

Juice the carrots, lime, cantaloupe, and pineapple. Add the remaining ingredients to the juice and blend until smooth.

Refresh

. . . .

1/2 small watermelon (remove rind)

5 sprigs mint

Pinch of Himalayan sea salt

Stevia, to taste (optional)

Juice the melon (with its rind) and mint; stir in the remaining ingredients to taste.

Replenish

. . . .

1/4 whole pineapple, peeled and cored

1 inch unpeeled gingerroot

1 lime, peeled

1/2 mango, skin and pit removed

8–10 ounces coconut water

1/4 teaspoon ground turmeric

Juice the pineapple, ginger, and lime, then combine with the mango, coconut water, and turmeric. Blend until smooth.

Elixirs for Great Skin

Skin So Soft

. . . .

8 ounces coconut water

Pinch of chamomile tea

1/4 cantaloupe, rind and seeds removed

2 ounces rose hip oil

1/2 quince (or green apple)

1 Meyer lemon, peeled

1 teaspoon maqui berry powder

Combine all the ingredients in a blender. Blend until smooth.

Green Goddess

. . . .

3 medium cucumbers (with skins)

¼ clove garlic

2 sprigs parsley

1 cup spinach

2 lemons, peeled

½ avocado, peeled and pitted

1 teaspoon flax oil

¼ Serrano chile

1 tablespoon apple cider vinegar

Pinch of pink Himalayan salt

Juice the cucumbers, garlic, parsley, spinach, and lemons. Combine with the remaining ingredients and blend until smooth.

BLENDER RECIPE: Add 6 ounces coconut water. Peel the cucumbers and squeeze the lemons by hand. Blend all the ingredients until smooth.

Cure for the Common Cold

Feel Better

. . . .

3 oranges, peeled

2 lemons, peeled

1 inch unpeeled gingerroot

1 cup coconut water

1 tablespoon apple cider vinegar

Pinch of cayenne

1 tablespoon honey (try raw honey for deeper flavor and higher antioxidant content)

1 sprig thyme, for garnish

Juice the citrus and ginger. Combine with the coconut water, vinegar, cayenne, and honey in a blender; blend until smooth. Garnish with fresh thyme. Heat for a warm, healing elixir.

BLENDER RECIPE: Peel the oranges and squeeze the lemons by hand. Blend all the ingredients until smooth.

Thirst Quenchers

Fresh

· · · · · · · · · · · · · · · · · · · ·

2 Meyer lemons, peeled

12–16 ounces unsweetened coconut water

$\frac{1}{4}$ cup sparkling water (optional)

Juice the lemons and combine with the coconut water. Add the sparkling water for extra zing!

BLENDER RECIPE: Hand-squeeze the lemons and blend with the coconut water.

Summer Quench

· · · · · · · · · · · · · · · · · · · ·

$\frac{1}{2}$ small watermelon (remove rind)

1 lime

Coconut water from 1 young coconut or 3-4 ounces of coconut water

Juice the watermelon and lime. Combine with the coconut water.

BLENDER RECIPE: Remove the watermelon rind and squeeze the lime by hand. Blend all the ingredients until smooth.

More Detoxifying Morning Elixirs

South Pacific

· · · · · · · · · · · · · · · · · · · ·

$\frac{1}{2}$ whole pineapple, peeled and cored

2 oranges, peeled

2 inches lemongrass

1 inch unpeeled gingerroot

$\frac{1}{4}$ teaspoon ground turmeric

4-6 ounces water

Juice all the ingredients except the water. Then add the water to the juice.

BLENDER RECIPE: Peel the oranges and peel and grate the ginger. Blend all the ingredients until smooth.

Citrus Singe

2 oranges, peeled

½ cup raspberries

Dash of vanilla extract

¼ teaspoon cinnamon

Pinch of ground habanero chile

6–8 ounces water

Juice the oranges. Combine all the ingredients in a blender and blend until smooth.

BLENDER RECIPE: Peel and juice the oranges by hand and blend all the ingredients until smooth.

Brighten Up

¾ honeydew melon (remove rind and seeds)

1 lemon, peeled

½ inch unpeeled gingerroot

1 tablespoon apple cider vinegar

Pinch of cayenne pepper

Stevia, to taste (optional)

Juice the melon, lemon, and ginger. Stir in the vinegar, cayenne, and stevia to taste.

More Afternoon and Evening Juice Therapy

Melon Mint Greens

1 medium cucumber (with skin)

1 small watermelon, rind removed

1 cup spinach

3 green leaf lettuce leaves

2 limes, peeled

4 sprigs mint

Juice all the ingredients.

Crimson Thirst

2 carrots

½ medium raw beet

2 medium cucumbers (with skins)

1 cup spinach

3 stalks celery

2 lemons, peeled

Juice all the ingredients.

Hearty Harvest

··················

1/2 whole pineapple, peeled and cored

2 medium cucumbers (with skins)

3 green leaf lettuce leaves

1/2 whole bok choy

1/4 bunch watercress

2 limes, peeled

1/2 avocado

Juice all the ingredients except the avocado. Blend the juice with the avocado.

Sweet Kick

··················

2 Pink Lady apples

1 1/2 medium cucumbers

2 stalks celery

1 green chard leaf

1 cup spinach

3 sprigs parsley

1 inch unpeeled gingerroot

1 lemon, peeled

Juice all the ingredients.

Leafy Citrus Blend

··················

1 medium cucumber (with skin)

2 stalks celery

1 grapefruit, peel removed

1 lemon, peel removed

3 green leaf lettuce leaves

1/2 cup spinach

2 leaves kale

3–4 sprigs mint

2–3 sprigs cilantro

Stevia, to taste

Juice all the ingredients.

European

··················

2 Granny Smith apples

1/2 medium cucumber

2 stalks celery

2 leaves kale

2 leaves collard greens

3 sprigs parsley

1 small sprig oregano

2 lemons, peel removed

Juice all the ingredients.

Mountain Magic

• • • • • • • • • • • • • • • • • • •

3 lemons, peel removed

½ cup blueberries

1 tablespoon chia seeds

Maple syrup, to taste

Pinch of cayenne

8–10 ounces water

Juice the lemons, then combine the remaining ingredients and blend until smooth.

Spice It Up

• • • • • • • • • • • • • • • • • • •

2 Granny Smith apples

1 medium cucumber (with skin)

2 stalks celery

1 cup spinach

½ inch unpeeled gingerroot

1 inch lemongrass

¼ cup cilantro

¼ serrano chile (seeds optional)

Juice all the ingredients.

Sweet Superfood Milk Shakes

Peach Cobbler

• • • • • • • • • • • • • • • • • • •

2 Fuji apples

1 peach

6 ounces walnut milk (directions below)

2 tablespoons gluten-free oats

½ teaspoon cinnamon

Maple syrup, to taste

Juice the apples. Combine the peaches, walnut milk, oats, and cinnamon with the apple juice. Blend, sweetening with maple syrup to taste.

WALNUT MILK: Soak 1 cup of walnuts in filtered water overnight. Blend soaked walnuts with 4 cups water. Strain the mixture through a nut milk bag to remove the nut pulp.

Walnut Cookies

· · · · · · · · · · · · · · · · ·

4 pears

½ cup black walnut husk tea (directions below)

¼ cup black walnuts

2 tablespoons gluten-free oats

2 dates, pitted

Maple syrup, to taste (optional)

Juice the pears. Add the juice to the walnut tea, walnuts, oats, and dates. Blend, adding maple syrup to taste.

BLACK WALNUT HUSK TEA: Soak 1 cup black walnut husks in 4 cups filtered water overnight. In the morning, strain and reserve the liquid.

Tropical Julius

· · · · · · · · · · · · · · · · ·

3 medium carrots

2 oranges, peel removed

¼ cup cubed pineapple

1 lime, peel removed

¼ cup cubed mango

¼ cup coconut milk

4 Brazil nuts

Dash of vanilla extract

Nutmeg, for garnish

Juice the carrots, oranges, pineapple, and lime. Combine the juice with the mango, coconut milk, Brazil nuts, and vanilla; blend until smooth. Garnish with a sprinkle of nutmeg.

Blueberry Pie

. . . .

1/2 lemon, peel removed

8–10 ounces pecan milk (directions below)

1/4 cup full-fat canned coconut milk

1/2 cup blueberries

1 teaspoon chia seeds

1 teaspoon golden flaxseeds

1/4 teaspoon vanilla extract

Honey, to taste

Juice the lemon. Combine the juice with the pecan milk, coconut milk, blueberries, chia seeds, flaxseeds, and vanilla. Blend all the ingredients until smooth, sweetening with honey to taste.

PECAN MILK: Soak 1 cup pecans overnight in filtered water. In the morning, combine the nuts with 16 ounces water in a blender; blend thoroughly. Strain the mixture through a nut milk bag to remove the nut pulp.

Vanilla Spiced Crème

. . . .

10-12 ounces macadamia nut milk (directions below)

1/2 banana

1/4 cup canned coconut milk

1/4 teaspoon vanilla extract

Pinch of nutmeg

Pinch of allspice

1/2 teaspoon cinnamon

Maple syrup, to taste

Combine all the ingredients (except the maple syrup) and blend until smooth. Sweeten to taste.

MACADAMIA NUT MILK: Soak 1 cup of macadamia nuts overnight in filtered water. In the morning, blend with 32 ounces of filtered water and strain through a nut milk bag to remove the nut pulp.

Monkey Treat

· · · · · · · · · · · · · · · ·

1 tablespoon almond butter

⅛ cup cacao powder

4–6 Medjool dates, pitted

½ cup young coconut meat or ½ cup coconut milk

½ banana

8–10 ounces coconut water

Combine all the ingredients in a blender and blend until smooth.

Lava Flow

· · · · · · · · · · · · · · · ·

1 lemon, peel removed

8–10 ounces almond milk

¼ cup young coconut meat or ¼ cup full-fat coconut milk

½ cup strawberries

¼ cup raspberries

⅛ cup cherries (pitted)

Dash of vanilla extract

Honey, to taste

Juice the lemon. Combine the lemon juice with the remaining ingredients (except the honey) in a blender, and blend until smooth. Sweeten with honey to taste.

Suja Spirits

Glowing Margagreena

· · · · · · · · · · · · · · · ·

2 ounces Apple Greens juice (recipe follows)

1 ounce freshly squeezed orange juice

2 ounces tequila

Ice, as desired

Crunchy sea salt, for rim of glass (optional)

Lime wedge, for garnish

Juice the Apple Greens ingredients and mix 2 ounces with the orange juice. Combine the juices with tequila and ice in a cocktail shaker. Shake until thoroughly mixed. If you like, wet the rim of a glass and place the glass top-side down in a dish filled with sea salt to coat the rim. Add a lime wedge for garnish.

Makes 1

Apple Greens

· · · · · · · · · · · · · · · · ·

2 Granny Smith apples

2 celery stalks

1 medium cucumber (with skin)

2 sprigs parsley

1 cup spinach

2 leaves kale

½ green bell pepper, seeds removed

2 lemons, peel removed

Juice all the ingredients.

Makes 14–16 ounces

Ruby Rush

· · · · · · · · · · · · · · · ·

4 ounces Life Line juice (recipe follows)

2 ounces gin

1 ounce Campari

5 ounces sweet vermouth

Ice, as desired

1 small cucumber, thinly sliced, for garnish

Juice the Life Line ingredients and combine 4 ounces with the gin, Campari, vermouth, and ice in a cocktail shaker. Shake until thoroughly mixed. Pour into a glass, add a cucumber slice on top for garnish.

Life Line

· · · · · · · · · · · · · · · ·

2 carrots

1 apple

½ medium raw unpeeled beet

1 medium cucumber (with skin)

½ teaspoon ground turmeric

Juice all the ingredients.

Makes 14–16 ounces

Simply Refreshing

. . . .

2 ounces Arise juice (recipe follows)

2 ounces vodka

Ice, as desired

1 orange, sliced thinly, for garnish

Juice the Arise juice ingredients and combine with vodka and ice in a cocktail shaker. Shake until thoroughly mixed. Pour into a glass and garnish with 1 or 2 thin orange slices.

Arise

. . . .

4 oranges, peel removed

$1/4$ whole pineapple, peeled and cored

$1/2$ cup basil

Pinch of cardamom powder

Pinch of cayenne powder

4-6 ounces water

Juice the fruit and basil. Stir in the cardamom, cayenne, and water.

Makes 12–14 ounces

ACKNOWLEDGMENTS

· ·

We wrote *The Suja Juice Solution* to give readers easy access to lifelong healthy eating habits by combining nutrient-dense juice and whole-food meals, and we didn't do it alone! This book wouldn't be complete without a thank-you to the many contributors who brought this program to life.

First and foremost, we would like to thank our extraordinary writing and book team beginning with Josh Goldin, our investor and great friend, who is responsible for getting this whole project rolling. Thank you, Josh, for connecting us with our wonderful agent Yfat Reiss Gendell at Foundry Literary + Media. Yfat—we feel so fortunate to have been connected with you. Along with your brilliant team, you saw the value of our message and worked tirelessly to introduce the Suja lifestyle to the world. Many thanks to executive assistant Amanda Brozman and the Foundry foreign rights and finance teams that include Kirsten Neuhaus, Jessica Regel, Sara DeNobrega, and Michon Vanderpoel. You have all played an instrumental part in this wild process and held our hands every step of the way. We couldn't have picked a better literary team, and we thank you deeply for turning our vision into a beautiful reality.

Next, we cannot express enough thanks to our co-writer and honorary Suja family member, Samantha Rose. Her tireless collaboration on this book and her great care in the delivery of our message has been tremendous. It has been a privilege to work with someone so talented, creative, and relentless. *No* is not a word in Samantha's vocabulary; despite a very ambitious time line and many, many changes, she smiled and said yes every step of the way. We could not be more grateful for her involvement.

We feel truly blessed to have found the perfect home for this book with Grand Central Publishing. We owe a huge thank-you to our incredible editor Sarah Pelz, whose wisdom, flexibility, and belief in our project made us feel right at home. Thank you also to Morgan Hedden for all of your behind-the-scenes help. We're beyond grateful to the support of the entire Grand Central

Publishing team, including Jamie Raab, Deb Futter, Karen Murgolo, Brian McLendon, and Amanda Pritzker. We owe a huge thank-you to Matthew Ballast and Bobbilyn Jones for their tireless work to get us publicity for the book. We also have to thank Rick Cobban in sales, who helped us explore every angle for distribution, and Yasmin Mathew, who kept the manuscript, book design, and book production on track. Without this exceptional team, this book would not be possible. *Thank you* feels like an insufficient expression of our gratitude for your guidance and expertise.

We owe another huge hug of gratitude to our Suja family. We love you more than we can say! You all have individually and collectively shaped Suja into the unique, once-in-a-lifetime experience we are privileged to be a part of every single day. We are humbled and beyond grateful to be in this together with you. Without all of your hard work, creativity, dedication, and support day after day, Suja would not be what it is.

Our warmest thanks to Eric Ethans, "the raw food guy," juice visionary, and co-founder of Suja. We are blessed to have you as our partner and friend. Your juice is magic and your creativity is unmatched. Your passion for and dedication to organic food has inspired us to create products of the highest quality. Also a great big thank-you to James Brennan, who has always pushed the envelope to make Suja be all that it can be. James inspires all of us to dream big. Finally, a special thanks to Bryan Riblett, Suja's chief juicer. Not only are your culinary instincts always spot-on, but your insatiable work ethic is something to be marveled at.

Finally, this book wouldn't have found a home at all without the loyal Suja customers who have believed in us, trusted us, and cheered us on through our growth from a small San Diego home delivery service into a nationally distributed brand. Without you, none of this would be possible. We are eternally grateful for your unwavering support in our mission to put simple, pure, and transparent products into as many hands as possible. It is because of you that we are able to do what we love every day!

CONVERTING TO METRICS

Volume Measurement Conversions

U.S.	METRIC
¼ teaspoon	1.25 ml
½ teaspoon	2.5 ml
¾ teaspoon	3.75 ml
1 teaspoon	5 ml
1 tablespoon	15 ml
¼ cup	62.5 ml
½ cup	125 ml
¾ cup	187.5 ml
1 cup	250 ml

Weight Conversion Measurements

U.S.	METRIC
1 ounce	28.4 g
8 ounces	227.5 g
16 ounces (1 pound)	455 g

Cooking Temperature Conversions

CELSIUS/CENTIGRADE	0°C and 100°C are arbitrarily placed at the melting and boiling points of water and standard to the metric system
FAHRENHEIT	Fahrenheit established 0°F as the stabilized temperature when equal amounts of ice, water, and salt are mixed

To convert temperatures in Fahrenheit to Celsius, use this formula:

$$C = (F - 32) \times 0.5555$$

So, for example, if you are baking at 350°F and want to know that temperature in Celsius, use this calculation:

$$C = (350 - 32) \times 0.5555 = 176.66°C$$

HOW SUJA IS MADE

· ·

Every one of our juices is made to order—in fact, *we're farm-to-bottle-to-shelves in just 8 days!* We value sourcing local ingredients and do so whenever possible. Our primary produce distribution supplier and partner—Jack Family Farms—provides a majority of the freshly harvested fruits and vegetables used to create our cold-pressured juices. We joined forces in 2013 under one cohesive business to allow us to better manage production from farm to bottle. We make our juices using cold pressure (also known as high-pressure processing or HPP) to destroy pathogens while preserving vitamins, enzymes, and nutrients. The result is better-tasting, more colorful juice that has better nutrient retention than juices made with alternative processes that use heat to destroy pathogens.

Please visit coldpressured.org to learn more about high-pressure processing. All Suja juices and smoothies are certified USDA Organic, Non-GMO, Kosher, and Gluten Free.

ABOUT THE SUJA FAMILY

Suja is now the fastest-growing organic, cold-pressed, and non-GMO beverage company in the United States. In 2014 *Forbes* magazine ranked Suja as the third most promising company in America. Whole Foods Markets awarded Suja its Supplier of the Year Award for 2013. Suja prides itself in making the highest-quality products that are all organic, non-GMO, and utilize an innovative technology called high hydrostatic pressure processing or HPP to ensure product safety and retention of essential vitamins and nutrients.

Suja was founded by four diverse San Diegans from different walks of life who came together because of a shared dream to help people everywhere transform their lives through conscious nutrition.

ANNIE LAWLESS, co-founder of Suja Juice and creator of all original meal recipes in the program, is the primary voice of *The Suja Juice Solution*, sharing her extensive knowledge of health and wellness with readers— and most important, her enthusiasm. Annie embodies Suja's vision of healthy eating for a long, beautiful life and brings years of experience in holistic nutrition to every aspect of the company. A certified holistic health coach (CHHC), Annie studied the health benefits of dietary and physical influences on the body and mind at the Institute for Integrative Nutrition. She developed a passion for nutrition at a young age after years of managing her own food sensitivities and celiac disease. She saw her health vastly improve when she began juicing following her own modified organic diet. When not in the kitchen, Annie practices yoga daily and travels the country spearheading consumer education for Suja.

JEFF CHURCH, co-founder and CEO of Suja Juice, balanced the many demands involved with building the fastest growing cold-pressed-juice business in America with the opportunity to help develop and introduce *The Suja Juice Solution* to readers. A successful social entrepreneur, Jeff earned an MBA at Harvard Business School and a BA from Michigan State University. Jeff is also the co-founder of Nika Water, which donates 100 percent of its profits to bring clean water to those without it in developing areas of the world. When he's not at the office, Jeff enjoys running, climbing, and most recently yoga. He has run in more than 50 marathons and five ultramarathons, and has climbed five of the seven summits—the highest mountains on the seven continents. He lives in San Diego with his wife of 25 years, Linda, and their four children.

JAMES BRENNAN, born and raised in Rockaway Beach (Queens), New York, is the managing partner of San Diego's Enlightened Hospitality Group, the innovative group that introduced the concept of "social dining" that has spread nationwide. Brennan and his team transformed dining out, making dinner not just a meal, but a complete experience—combining dining with nightlife in his award-winning, fabric-inspired restaurants, Searsucker and Herringbone. While looking for a way to get healthy and keep up with his wife and four children, Brennan tried Suja Juice in its earliest development. After his first taste, Brennan knew the juice could help improve people's health and led Suja's entrance into the marketplace.

ERIC ETHANS, co-founder and director of development of Suja Juice, was born and raised in California, where he opened his first raw food restaurant at the age of 20 in San Diego. A world traveler, he worked in restaurants in Fiji, Australia, Bali, and New Zealand, chasing his dreams of surfing and working as a self-proclaimed nutritional chef. In 2007 he and Bryan Riblett opened an organic juice delivery service and restaurant called "blissful." It wasn't until five years later that Eric would meet Annie, Jeff, and James to create Suja.

BRYAN RIBLETT, VP of commercialization and chief innovation officer for Suja Juice, created every juice recipe for *The Suja Juice Solution* and leads the team in producing every SKU from scratch each week. Over the past two years Bryan developed over 35 organic, non-GMO beverages under three different product lines ranging from cold-pressed juices to smoothies, cold-brewed teas, and holiday items. Valedictorian of his graduating class at the Culinary Institute of America, Bryan enjoys not only transforming fresh produce into delicious beverages but cooking as well.

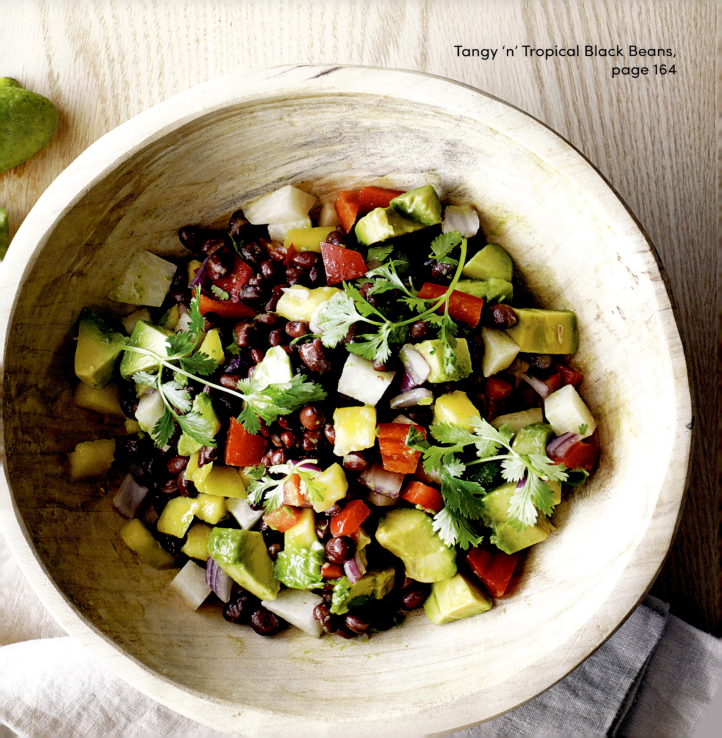

Tangy 'n' Tropical Black Beans,
page 164

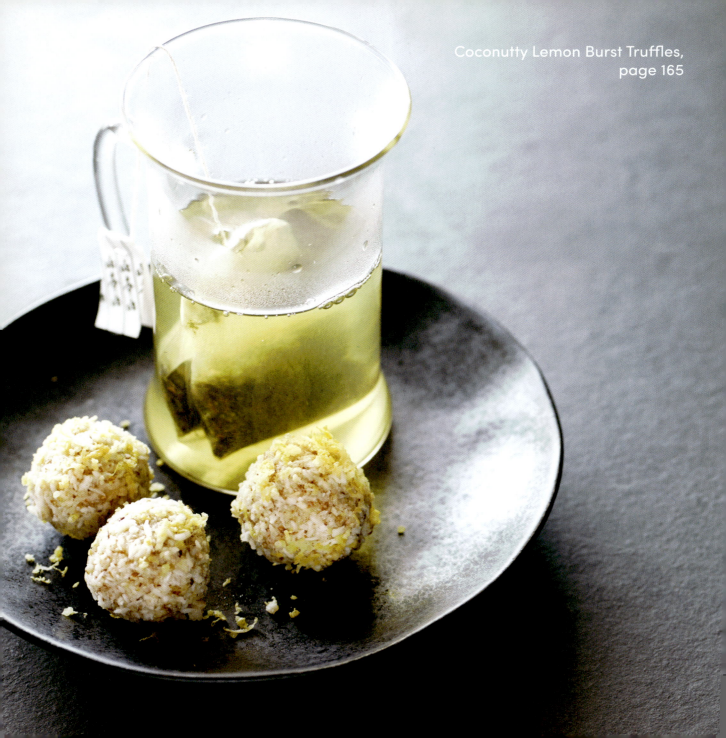

Coconutty Lemon Burst Truffles,
page 165

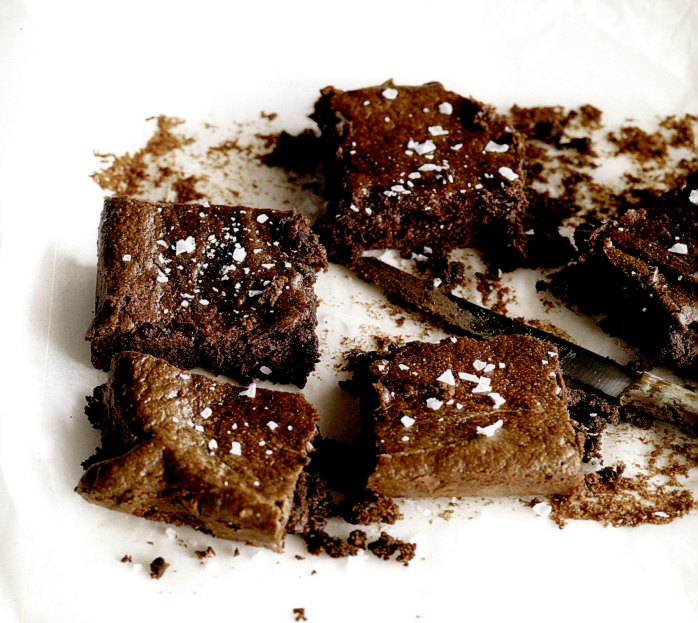

Brownies Done Better, page 165

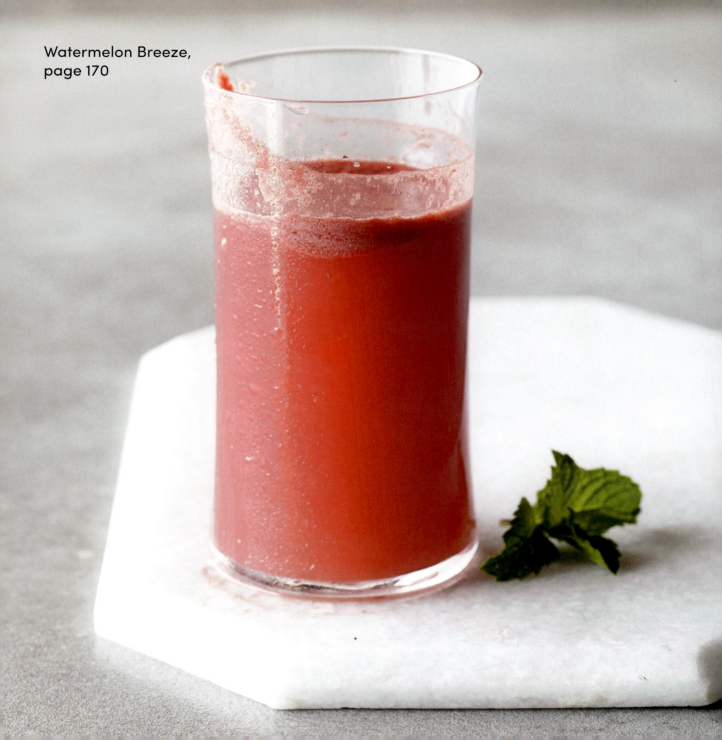

Watermelon Breeze,
page 170

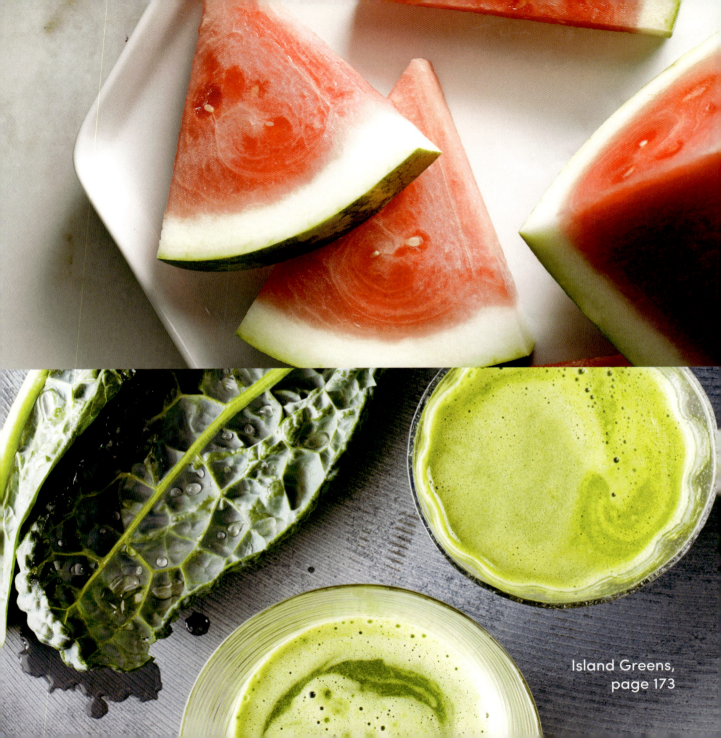

Island Greens,
page 173

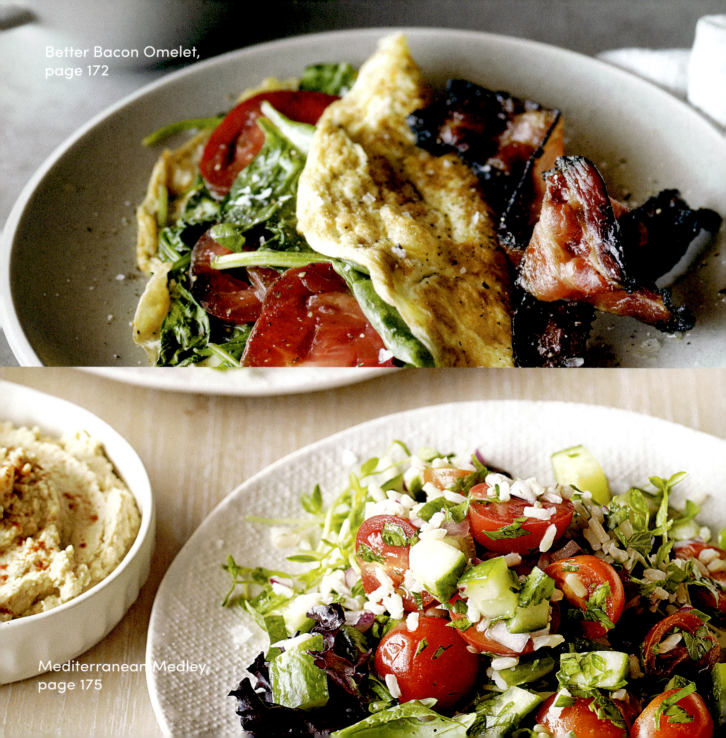

Better Bacon Omelet,
page 172

Mediterranean Medley,
page 175

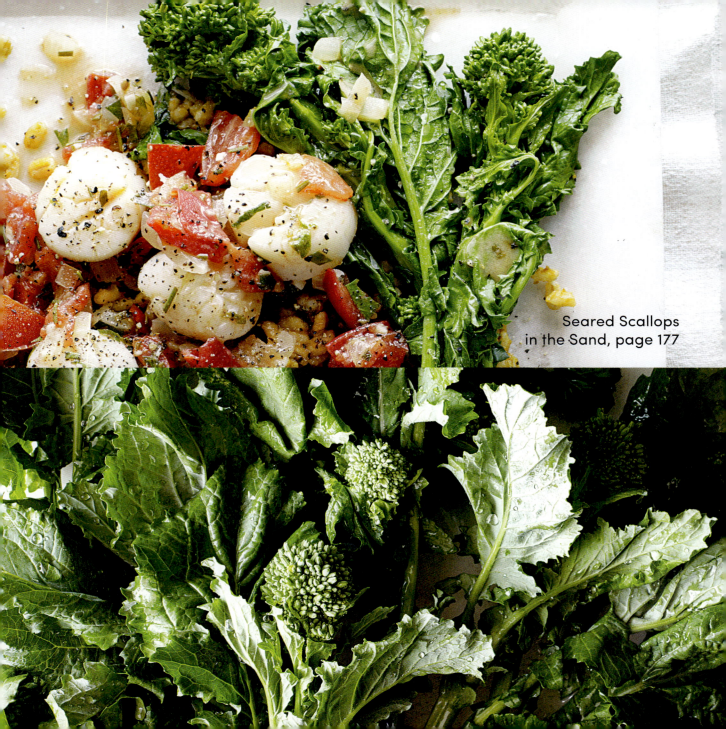

Seared Scallops
in the Sand, page 177

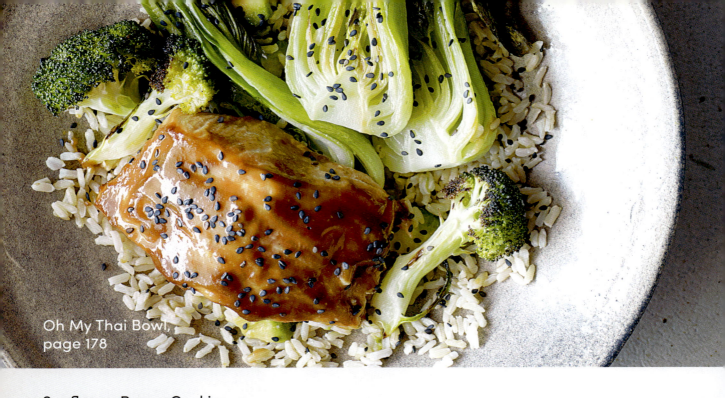

Oh My Thai Bowl,
page 178

Sunflower Power Cookies,
page 179

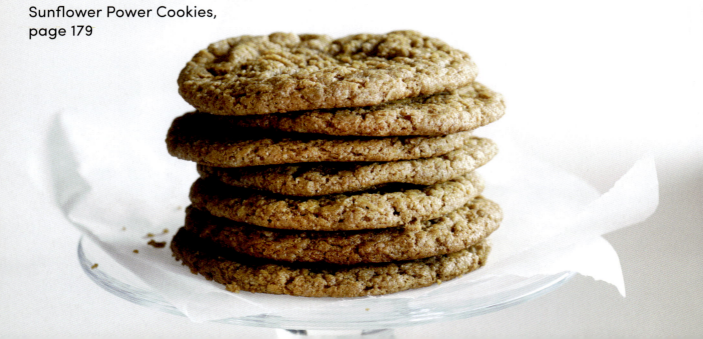

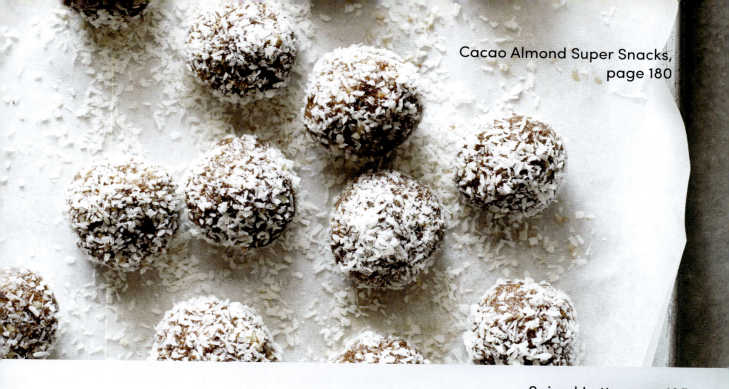

Cacao Almond Super Snacks, page 180

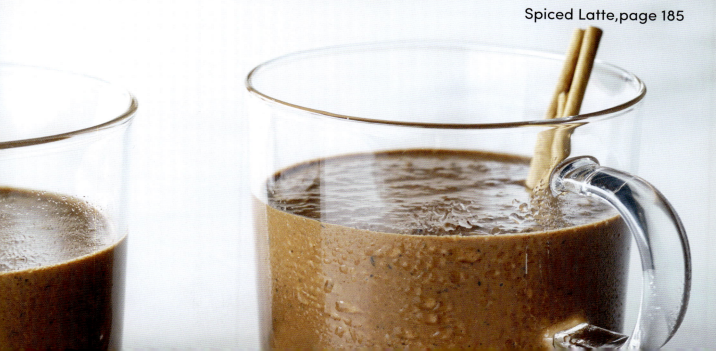

Spiced Latte, page 185

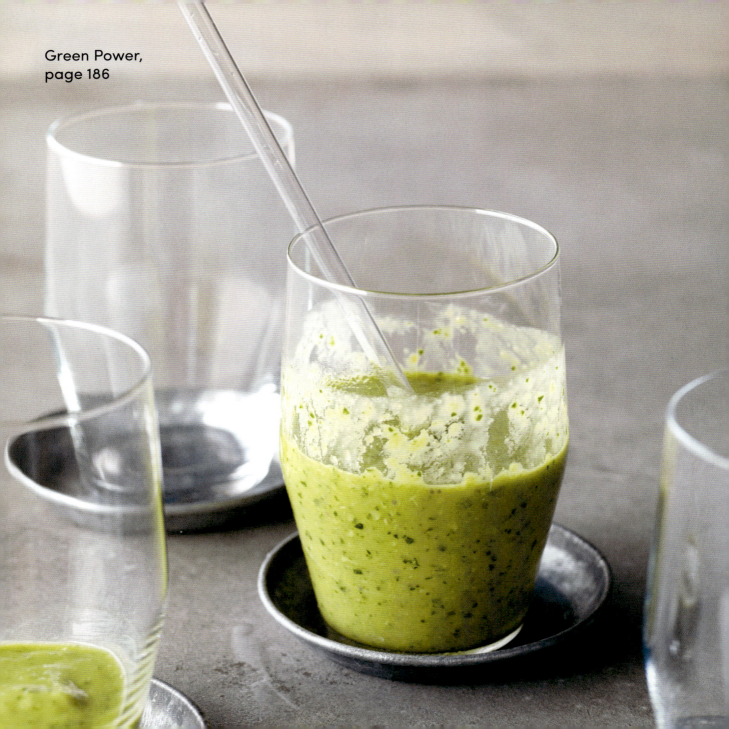

Green Power,
page 186

Replenish, page 188

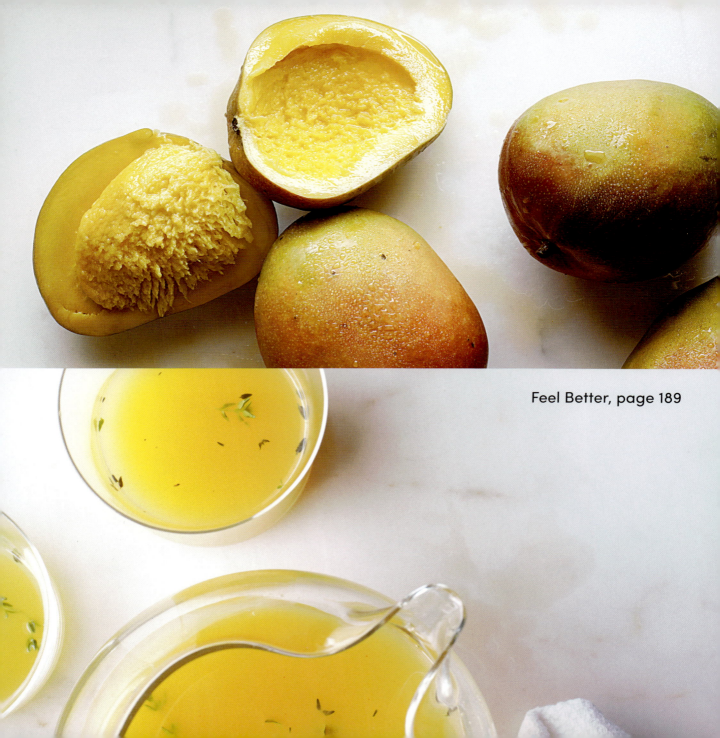

Feel Better, page 189

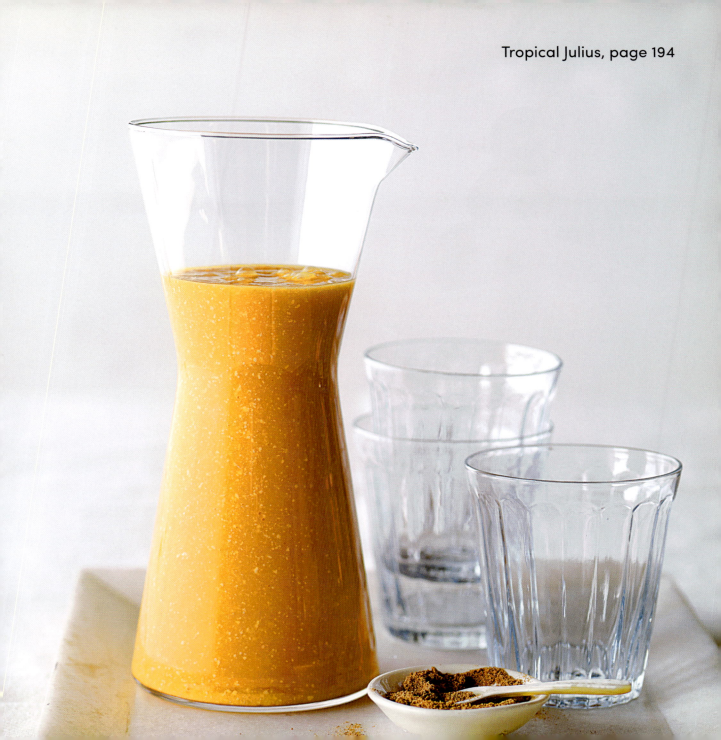

Tropical Julius, page 194

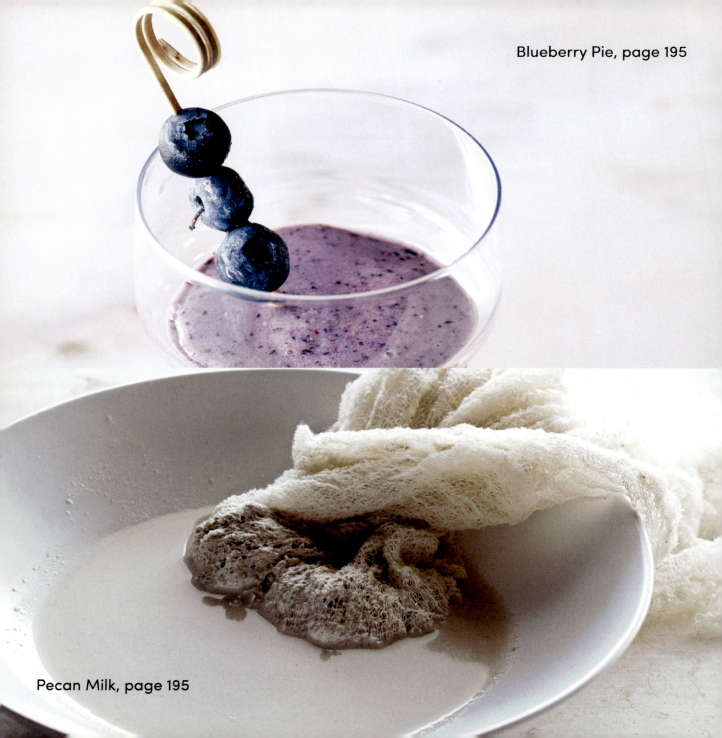

Blueberry Pie, page 195

Pecan Milk, page 195

REFERENCES

INTRODUCTION.
JUICE IS A LIFE CHANGER

Blake, Kati, and Dr. George Krucik. "Nutritional Deficiencies (Malnutrition)." *Healthline*. July 26, 2012. http://www.healthline.com/health/malnutrition#Overview1.

Cross, Joe. "Making Fresh Juice a Part of a Well-Balanced, Plant-Based Diet Is an Important Tool for Achieving Good Health." *Reboot with Joe*. http://www.rebootwithjoe.com/juicing/benefits.

"Diseases and Conditions: Celiac." Mayo Clinic. http://www.mayoclinic.org/diseases-conditions/celiac-disease/basics/definition/con-20030410.

Egan, Carol. "Non-Negotiable #14, Juicing." *It's Not About Food*. http://carol-egan.com/blog/page/2.

Kellow, Juliette. "Dieting and Metabolism." *Dietitian*. http://www.weightlossresources.co.uk/calories/burning_calories/starvation.htm.

Myers, Leslie. "Juicing 101: Benefits, Ingredients and Recipes." *Competitor*. May 8, 2014. http://running.competitor.com/2014/05/nutrition/juicing-101-benefits-ingredients-recipes_102219.

"Natural Tips for Boosting Your Metabolism." Global Healing Center. http://www.globalhealingcenter.com/natural-health/tips-for-boosting-your-metabolism.

"Symptoms of Eczema." National Eczema Foundation. http://nationaleczema.org/eczema/symptoms.

Thompson, Laura. "Monster Cravings Caused by Simple Nutrient Deficiencies." Southern California Institute of Clinical Nutrition. http://www.scicn.com/article-monstercravings.html.

Valliant, Melissa. "Do Juice Cleanses Work? 10 Truths About the Fad." *Huffington Post*. http://www.huffingtonpost.ca/2012/03/22/do-juice-cleanses-work_n_1372305.html.

Watson, Dr. Lisa. "Nutrient Deficiencies in Celiac Disease." Dr. Lisa Watson. http://www.drlisawatson.com/nutrient-deficiencies-celiac.

Zuckerbot, Tanya. "3 Things to Know Before Starting a Juice Cleanse." Fox News. May 20, 2014. http://www.foxnews.com/health/2014/05/20/3-things-to-know-before-starting-juice-cleanse-for-weight-loss.

CHAPTER 1. THE SCIENCE BEHIND THE SUJA JUICE SOLUTION

"4 Main Nutrition Principles." Amherst College. https://www.amherst.edu/athletics/department/strength/nutrition.

Amidor, Toby. "Unraveling Natural vs. Added Sugar." *Toby Amidor Nutrition*. February 7, 2012. http://tobyamidornutrition.com/2012/02/unraveling-natural-vs-added-sugar.

Bardot, J. B. "12 Easy Ways to Remove Acid Buildup from Your Body, Alkalize Your pH, and Beat Disease." *Natural News*. January 19, 2013. http://www.naturalnews.com/038749_alkalize_ph_balance_disease_prevention.html.

Blauer, Stephen. *The Juicing Book*. New York: Avery, 1989.

Bosely, Sarah. "Sugar, Not Fat, Exposed as Deadly Villain in Obesity Epidemic." *The Guardian*. March 20, 2013. http://www.theguardian.com/society/2013/mar/20/sugar-deadly-obesity-epidemic.

Bridgeford, Ross. "Health Benefits of Liquid Chlorophyll." *Alkaline Diet Blog*. http://www.energiseforlife.com/wordpress/2009/02/11/health-benefits-of-liquid-chlorophyll.

Canole, Drew. "Juice to Break Free of Sugar Addiction." Fitlife.tv. July 11, 2013. http://fitlife.tv/juice-to-break-free-of-sugar-addiction.

"Cold Press vs. Centrifugal Juicers." Vive Juicery. http://vivejuicery.com/pages/cold-pressed-vs-centrifugal.

Coull, Bruce M. "Inflammation and Stroke." American Stroke Association. http://stroke.ahajournals.org/content/38/2/631.full.

"Enzymes: The Fountain of Vibrant Life." The Living Centre. http://www.thelivingcentre.com/cms/body/enzymes-the-fountain-of-vibrant-life.

Fagley, Heidi. "Juice to Boost Immunity—Fight the Flu with Fruits and Veggies." *Natural News*. January 25, 2011. http://www.naturalnews.com/031099_juicing_immunity.html.

"Food Cravings: When Your Body Craves Certain Foods, It Is Actually Looking for Nutrients." Naturopathy Works Primary Care Clinic. http://natureworksbest.com/naturopathy-works/food-cravings.

Hari, Vani. "There's Proof: Processed Foods Are Harder to Digest." *Food Babe*. http://foodbabe.com/2012/08/01/theres-proof-processed-foods-are-harder-to-digest.

Hayes, Donald L. "Acid/Alkaline Balance." Greens First. http://www.greensfirst.com/gestion/acid-alkaline-balance.pdf.

"Inflammation and Heart Disease." American Heart Association. Updated July 29, 2014. http://www.heart.org/HEARTORG/Conditions/Inflammation-and-Heart-Disease_UCM_432150_Article.jsp.

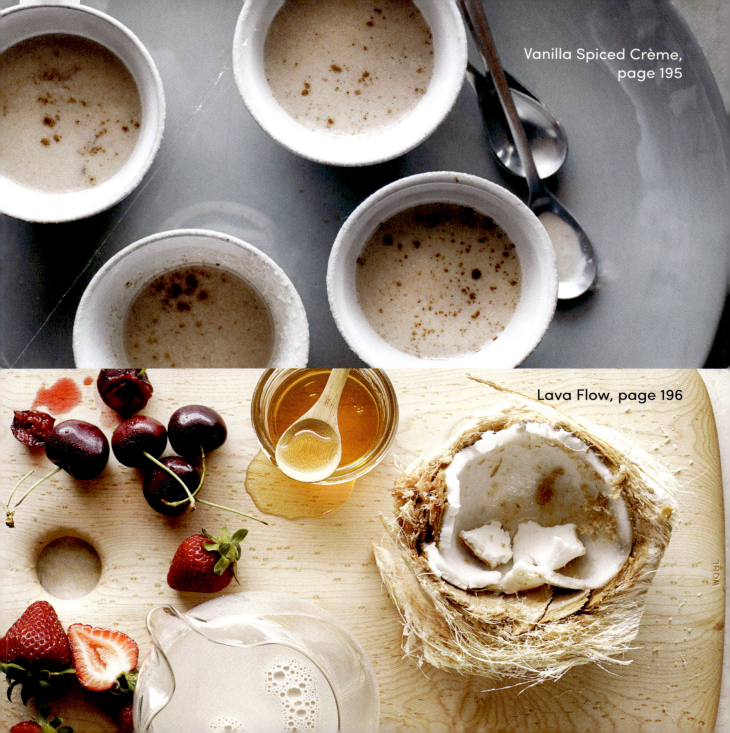

Vanilla Spiced Crème,
page 195

Lava Flow, page 196

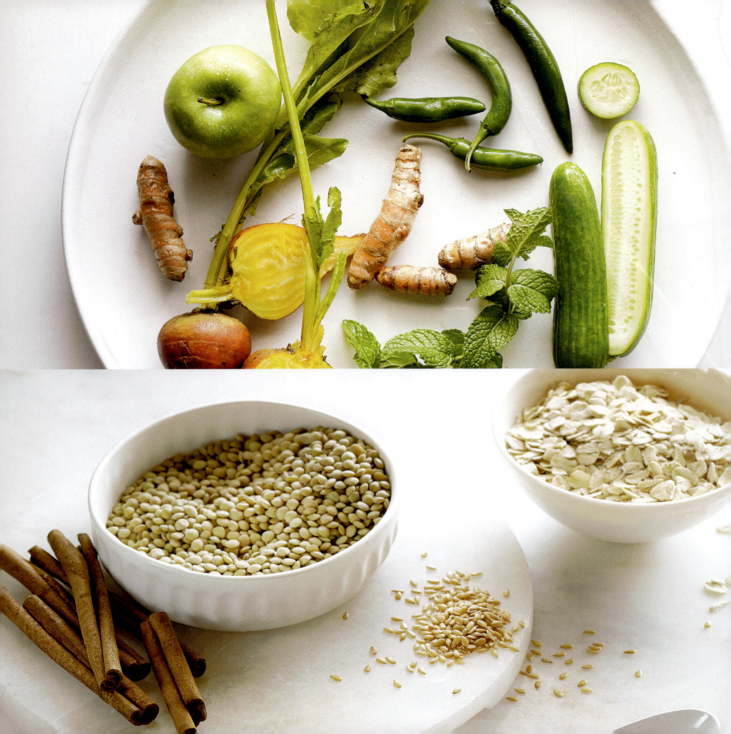

"Is a Toxic Colon Making You Sick?" Ogden Colon Therapy. http://www.ogdencolonhydrotherapy.com/toxic-colon-making-you-sick.

"Juice Terminology: What Does 'Cold Pressed' Really Mean?" *Well + Good NYC*. http://wellandgood.com/2014/07/13/juice-terminology-what-does-cold-pressed-really-mean.

Kobayashi, Lindsay. "The Worst Thing You Can Eat Is Sugar." *Public Health Perspective*. January 13, 2014. http://blogs.plos.org/publichealth/2014/01/13/worst-sugar.

"Macronutrients: The Importance of Carbohydrate, Protein, and Fat." McKinley Health Center. http://www.mckinley.illinois.edu/handouts/macronutrients.htm.

Marchese, Dr. Marianne. "Colon Cancer: Which Toxins or Chemicals Cause This?" *EmpowHER*. http://www.empowher.com/colorectal-cancer/content/colon-cancer-which-toxins-or-chemical-cause-dr-marchese-video.

Marquis, Dr. David M. "How Inflammation Affects Every Aspect of Your Health." Mercola. http://articles.mercola.com/sites/articles/archive/2013/03/07/inflammation-triggers-disease-symptoms.aspx.

McEvoy, Michael. "The Electrolyte Solution: Saving Your Cells from Dehydration." *Metabolic Healing*. September 14, 2011. http://metabolichealing.com/the-electrolyte-solution-saving-your-cells-from-dehydration.

Mercola, Dr. "Juicing: How Healthy Is It?" Mercola. April 19, 2014. http://articles.mercola.com/sites/articles/archive/2014/04/19/juicing-benefits.aspx.

Mercola, Dr. "What Are the Health Benefits of Carrots?" Mercola. December 28, 2013. http://articles.mercola.com/sites/articles/archive/2013/12/28/carrot-health-benefits.aspx.

Olivia, Fern. "5 Step Cleanse to Maximize Thyroid, Adrenal, Immune, and Digestive Health." MindBodyGreen. March 4, 2013. http://www.mindbodygreen.com/0-7920/5-step-cleanse-to-maximize-thyroid-adrenal-immune-digestive-health.html.

"Overview of the Digestive Process." Ivy Rose Holistic. September 10, 2014. http://www.ivy-rose.co.uk/HumanBody/Digestion/DigestiveSystem-BasicStages.php.

"Phytochemicals." American Cancer Society. http://www.cancer.org/treatment/treatmentsandsideeffects/complementaryandalternativemedicine/herbsvitaminsandminerals/phytochemicals.

"Phytonutrient Rich Foods: Add Color to Your Plate." Dana Farber/Brigham and Women's Cancer Center. https://www.dana-farber.org/uploadedFiles/Library/health-library/nutrition/phytonutrient-rich-foods.pdf.

"What Are Electrolytes?" *Medical News Today*. Updated November 9, 2013. http://www.medicalnewstoday.com/articles/153188.php.

"Why Your Cold Pressed Juice Is So Expensive." *Huffington Post*. March 7, 2014. http://www.huffingtonpost.com/2014/03/07/cold-pressed-juice_n_4911492.html.

Zimmerman, Maureen, and Beth Snow. "Nutrients Are Essential for Organ Function." *Essentials of Nutrition: A Functional Approach, v. 1.0*. http://catalog.flatworldknowledge.com/bookhub/reader/3728?e=zimmerman_1.0-ch03_s03.

CHAPTER 2. HOW THE SUJA JUICE SOLUTION WORKS

Coffman, Melodie Anne. "The Disadvantages of Dried Fruit." *SF Gate*. http://healthyeating.sfgate.com/disadvantages-dried-fruit-3227.html.

"The Dark Side of Caffeine." *Touchstone Essentials*. http://mytouchstoneessentials.com/the-dark-side-of-caffeine/#.U_WkuV7zopE.

Fallon, Sally, and Mary Enig. "Newest Research on Why You Should Avoid Soy." Mercola. http://www.mercola.com/article/soy/avoid_soy.htm.

"Fasting with Juice." Natural Health Techniques. http://naturalhealthtechniques.com/healingtechniquesjuice_fasting.htm.

Hendon, Jeremy. "10 Reasons to Avoid Eating Legumes." *Paleo Living Magazine*. http://paleomagazine.com/paleo-why-legumes-are-bad.

Hyman, Dr. Mark. "Dairy: 6 Reasons You Should Avoid It at All Costs." Dr. Mark Hyman. Updated June 24, 2010. http://drhyman.com/blog/2010/06/24/dairy-6-reasons-you-should-avoid-it-at-all-costs-2.

Hyman, Dr. Mark. "Eat Your Medicine." Dr. Mark Hyman. http://drhyman.com/downloads/eatyourmedicine.pdf.

"Is Deli Meat Paleo?" *Paleoista*. June 13, 2013. http://paleoista.com/news/is-deli-meat-paleo.

Melone, Linda. "10 Reasons to Stop Eating Red Meat." *Prevention*. http://www.prevention.com/food/healthy-eating-tips/10-reasons-stop-eating-red-meat?s=1.

Moyer, Melinda Wenner. "It's Time to End the War on Salt." *Scientific American*. July 8, 2011. http://www.scientificamerican.com/article/its-time-to-end-the-war-on-salt.

National Institute on Alcohol Abuse and Alcoholism. "Alcohol and Nutrition." *Alcohol Alert* 22. Updated October 2000. http://pubs.niaaa.nih.gov/publications/aa22.htm.

Sisson, Mark. "Why Grains Are Unhealthy." *Mark's Daily Apple*. November 5, 2013. http://www.marksdailyapple.com/why-grains-are-unhealthy/#axzz3B0gfl7q.

Stossel, Richard. "Why Hydrogenated Oils Should Be Avoided at All Costs." *Natural News*. November 04, 2008. http://www.naturalnews.com/024694_oil_food_oils.html.

Yan, Lin. "Dark Green Leafy Vegetables." U.S. Department of Agriculture. Last modified March 20, 2013. http://www.ars.usda.gov/News/docs .htm?docid=23199.

CHAPTER 3. THE IN AND OUT CROWD

"Alcohol and Nutrition." MedicineNet.com. http:// www.medicinenet.com/alcohol_and_nutrition/ page2.htm.

Allday, Erin. "Caffeine Dependence Tied to Physical, Emotional Problems." *SF Gate*. Updated March 5, 2014. http://www.sfgate.com/health/ article/Caffeine-dependence-tied-to-physical -emotional-5288887.php.

Atkins, Clyde. "7 Benefits of Almond Milk." EatGoodFood.org. August 20, 2013. http:// eatgoodfood.org/7-benefits-of-almond-milk.

Bruso, Jessica. "Does Stevia Affect Blood Sugar?" *SF Gate*. http://healthyeating.sfgate.com/stevia -affect-blood-sugar-7359.html.

Cassar, Allison. "Foods That Cause Bloating." Pure Inside Out. http://www.pureinsideout.com/foods -that-cause-bloating.html.

Chainani-Wu, Nita. "Safety and Anti-Inflammatory Activity of Curcumin: A Component of Turmeric." *Journal of Alternative and Complementary Medicine* 9, no. 1 (2003): 161–68.

Eaton, D. L., and J. D. Groopman. 1994. *The Toxicology of Aflatoxins*. New York: Academic Press, 1994, pp. 383–426.

"The Facts on Omega-3 Fatty Acids." *WebMD*. http://www.webmd.com/healthy-aging/ omega-3-fatty-acids-fact-sheet.

Fernandez, M. L. "Dietary Cholesterol Provided by Eggs and Plasma Lipoproteins in Healthy Populations." *Current Opinion in Clinical Nutrition and Metabolic Care* 9 (2006): 8–12.

Gates, Donna. "The Risks of Consuming Typical Grains & the Healthy Grains to Choose Instead." December 17, 2006. http://bodyecology .com/articles/risks_consuming_grains.php# .VA_UCl7zopE.

Gunnars, Kris. "Top 9 Reasons to Avoid Sugar as if Your Life Depended on It." *Authority Nutrition*. http://authoritynutrition .com/9-reasons-to-avoid-sugar.

Hartel, Kari. "Your Secret Weight-Loss Ingredient: Vinegar." *FitDay*. http://www.fitday.com/fitness -articles/nutrition/your-secret-weight-loss -ingredient-vinegar.html.

Harvard School of Public Health. "Obesity Prevention Source: Food and Diet." *Obesity Prevention Source*. http://www.hsph.harvard. edu/obesity-prevention-source/obesity-causes/ diet-and-weight.

Heathcote, J. G., and J. R. Hibbert. *Aflatoxins: Chemical and Biological Aspects*. New York: Elsevier, 1978, pp. 173–86.

Hu, F. B., M. J. Stampfer, E. B. Rimm, et al. "A Prospective Study of Egg Consumption and Risk of Cardiovascular Disease in Men and Women." *Journal of the American Medical Association* 281 (1999): 1387–94.

Hyman, Dr. Mark. "3 Hidden Ways Wheat Makes You Fat." Dr. Mark Hyman. Last updated January 25, 2013. http://drhyman.com/blog/2012/02/13/three-hidden-ways-wheat-makes-you-fat.

Hyman, Dr. Mark. "Are Your Food Allergies Making You Fat?" Dr. Mark Hyman. Last updated May 24, 2013. http://drhyman.com/blog/2010/04/20/are-your-food-allergies-making-you-fat.

Ireland, Corydon. "Hormones in Milk Can Be Dangerous." *Harvard University Gazette*. December 7, 2006. http://news.harvard.edu/gazette/2006/12.07/11-dairy.html.

Kauls, Nell. "5 Weight Loss Pitfalls and How to Avoid Them." *Nutritional Weight and Wellness*. http://www.weightandwellness.com/resources/articles-and-videos/weight-management-metabolism/5-weight-loss-pitfalls-and-how-to-avoid-them.

Khan, Alam, Mahpara Safdar, Mohammad Muzaffar Ali Khan, Khan Nawaz Khattak, and Richard A. Anderson. "Cinnamon Improves Glucose and Lipids of People with Type 2 Diabetes." American Diabetes Association. http://care.diabetesjournals.org/content/26/12/3215.full.

Korth, Christie. "Benefits of Dark Green Leafy Vegetables." Brain Balance Achievement Centers. March 2013. http://www.brainbalancecenters.com/blog/2013/03/healthy-bites-the-benefits-of-dark-green-leafy-vegetables.

Lawless, Annie. "The Guide to Healthy Oils." Suja Juice. http://www.sujajuice.com/blog/the-guide-to-healthy-oils.

Lawless, Annie. "Why Fats Are Phat." *Blawnde*. http://www.blawnde.com/fats-phat.

Lempert, Phil. "The 5 Things You Need to Know About Deli Meats." *Today*. Updated December 27, 2006. http://www.today.com/id/16361276/ns/today-today_food/t/things-you-need-know-about-deli-meats/#.VBBval7zopE.

Lewin, Jo. "The Health Benefits of…Coconut Milk." *BBC GoodFood*. http://www.bbcgoodfood.com/howto/guide/ingredient-focus-coconut-milk.

Liener, I. E. *Toxic Constituents of Plant Foodstuffs*. New York: Academic Press, 1969, pp. 392–94.

Melnick, Meredith. "Health Benefits of Eggs." *Huffington Post*. Updated March 30, 2013. http://www.huffingtonpost.com/2013/03/30/health-benefits-of-eggs-yolks_n_2966554.html.

Melone, Linda. "10 Reasons to Stop Eating Red Meat: It's Time to Unhand the Hamburger." *Prevention*. http://www.prevention.com/food/healthy-eating-tips/10-reasons-stop-eating-red-meat.

Mercola, Dr. "Agave Is Far Worse than High Fructose Corn Syrup." *Healthy Impact Daily News*. http://healthimpactnews.com/2013/agave-is-far-worse-than-high-fructose-corn-syrup.

Mercola, Dr. "Soy: This 'Miracle Health Food' Has Been Linked to Brain Damage and Breast Cancer." Mercola. September 18, 2010. http://articles.mercola.com/sites/articles/archive/2010/09/18/soy-can-damage-your-health.aspx.

Mercola, Dr. "The Health Dangers of Soy." *Huffington Post*. Updated October 23, 2012. http://www.huffingtonpost.com/dr-mercola/soy-health_b_1822466.html.

"Non-Starchy Veggies." Diabetes.co.uk. http://www.diabetes.co.uk/food/non-starchy-vegetables.html.

Orenstein, Beth W., and Dr. Lindsey Marcellin. "7 Foods That Spike Blood Sugar." *Everyday Health*. Last updated July 18, 2012. http://www.everydayhealth.com/type-2-diabetes-pictures/foods-that-spike-blood-sugar.aspx.

"Parsley Health Benefits." Natural Health Techniques. http://naturalhealthtechniques.com/diet_nutritionparsleybenefits.htm.

Repinski, Karyn. "How Sugar Ages Your Skin." *Prevention*. http://www.prevention.com/beauty/beauty/how-sugar-ages-your-skin.

Rocketto, Leah. "Dangerfood: Dried Fruit." *Greatist*. August 23, 2011. http://greatist.com/health/dangerfood-dried-fruit.

Rothman, Dr. Michael. "Why Fruit May Not Be So Good for You." MD Wellness. http://www.mdwellnessmd.com/wellness-information/why-fruit-may-not-be-so-good-for-you.

Terrain, Mary Vance. "The Dark Side of Soy." *Utne Reader*. August 2007. http://www.utne.com/science-and-technology/the-dark-side-of-soy.aspx.

"The Ugly Truth About Vegetable Oil." *Thank Your Body*. February 18, 2013. http://www.thankyourbody.com/vegetable-oils.

"What's Wrong with Beans and Legumes?" *Paleo Leap*. Last updated January 6, 2014. http://paleoleap.com/beans-and-legumes.

Yeager, Selene. "Protein: Your Secret Weight Loss Weapon." *Women's Health*. September 2, 2010. http://www.womenshealthmag.com/weight-loss/protein-weight-loss.

Young, Dr. Lisa. "Benefits of Nuts and Seeds." *Huffington Post*. Updated January 29, 2013. http://www.huffingtonpost.com/dr-lisa-young/healthy-foods_b_2115225.html.

CHAPTER 4. JUICY FAQ

Brooking, Katherine. "10 Foods That Sound Healthy (but Aren't)." *Cooking Light*. http://www.cookinglight.com/eating-smart/smart-choices/top-10-unhealthy-foods/energy-bars.

Cross, Joe. "Juice & Kids." *Reboot with Joe*. http://www.rebootwithjoe.com/kids/juice.

Dean, J., and P. Kendall. "Food Safety During Pregnancy." Colorado State University Extension. August 2012. http://www.ext.colostate.edu/pubs/foodnut/09372.html.

Georgiou, Claire. "What Do Your Food Cravings Really Mean?" *Reboot with Joe*. November 7, 2012. http://www.rebootwithjoe.com/what-do-your-food-cravings-really-mean.

"Glycemic index and glycemic load for 100+ foods." Harvard Health Publications. Harvard Medical School. http://www.health.harvard.edu/newsweek/Glycemic_index_and_glycemic_load_for_100_foods.htm.

"Glycemic Index." Center for Integrative Medicine, University of Wisconsin. http://www.amsa.org/healingthehealer/GlycemicIndex.pdf.

Gold, Mary V. "Organic Production/Organic Food: Information Access Tools." USDA National Agricultural Library. June 2007. http://www.nal.usda.gov/afsic/pubs/ofp/ofp.shtml.

Lipman, Dr. Frank. "7 Reasons Kale Is the New Beef." Dr. Frank Lipman. April 2004. http://www.drfranklipman.com/7-reasons-kale-is-the-new-beef.

"The Protein Myth." Physicians Committee for Responsible Medicine. http://pcrm.org/health/diets/vsk/vegetarian-starter-kit-protein.

Sears, Dr. Al. "Glycemic Index," Website, http://www.alsearsmd.com/glycemic-index.

Snyder, Kimberly. "The Difference in How Fructose and Glucose Affect Your Body." Kimberly Snyder. http://kimberlysnyder.net/blog/2012/04/14/the-difference-in-how-fructose-and-glucose-affect-your-body.

Sygo, Jennifer. "Your 'Eat More to Stay Fit for Life' Plan." *Oxygen Magazine*. September 2010. http://www.oxygenmag.com.au/Nutrition/tabid/620/entryid/1458/YOUR-EAT-MORE-TO-STAY-FIT-FOR-LIFE-PLAN.aspx.

"What about concerns of sugar in raw fruit juice?" Juice Press. FAQ. http://www.juicepress.com/sugar.

CHAPTER 5. YOUR NEW KITCHEN TOOLS

Cliver, Dean O. "Plastic and Wooden Cutting Boards." University of California–Davis Food Safety Laboratory. August 1, 2005. http://faculty.vetmed.ucdavis.edu/faculty/docliver/Research/cuttingboard.htm.

"Cold-Pressed Juice: The New Trend." *Body + Soul*. http://www.bodyandsoul.com.au/nutrition/nutrition+tips/cold+pressed+juice+the+new+trend,25495.

Heimer, Megan. "What's a Dehydrator, Why You Need One, How to Use It." LivingWhole.org. March 10, 2014. http://www.livingwhole.org/whats-a-dehydrator-why-you-need-one-how-to-use-it.

"Juicer Types: The Difference Between Cold Press Juicers vs. Centrifugal Juice Extractors." *Huffington Post*. Updated July 23, 2013. http://www.huffingtonpost.com/2013/02/08/juicer-types-cold-press_n_2618000.html.

Sellner, Jadah, and Jen Hansnard. "Juicing vs. Blending: What's the Difference?" Simple Green Smoothies. March 14, 2013. http://simplegreensmoothies.com/tips/juicing-vs-blending-whats-the-difference.

CHAPTER 6. GIVE YOURSELF A REVVING JUMP START

Corum, Cassandra. "Juicing 101: How to Ease Into and Out of a Cleanse." Active.com. http://www.active.com/nutrition/articles/juicing-101-how-to-ease-into-and-out-of-a-cleanse.

Felts, Lauren. "Is Green Juice the New Coffee?" The Holy Kale. http://www.theholykale.com/2013/01/is-green-juice-the-new-coffee.

Hose, Carl. "How to Detox Your Body." Gaiam Life. http://life.gaiam.com/article/how-detox-your-body.

"How Does Water Help Remove Harmful Toxins from Your Digestive Tract?" APEC Water. http://www.freedrinkingwater.com/water_health/health2/water-remove-harmful-toxins-from-digestive-tract.htm.

Lawless, Annie. "Organic Fresh Start." Suja Juice. http://www.sujajuice.com/wp-content/uploads/2014/03/Essentials_3Day_MealPlan-min.pdf.

McCluskey, Casey. "3 Healthy Ways to Kick Caffeine." MindBodyGreen. December 6, 2011. http://www.mindbodygreen.com/0-3604/3-Healthy-Ways-to-Kick-Caffeine.html.

CHAPTER 7. WEEK 1: 7 DAYS TO RESET

"6 Things You Don't Know About Kale." *Huffington Post*. Updated July 31, 2013. http://www.huffingtonpost.com/2013/07/30/kale-facts-nutrition-info_n_3671210.html.

Adams, Case. "Anti Diabetic Effects Found in Citrus Foods and Juices." Green Med Info. September 25, 2012. http://www.greenmedinfo.com/blog/anti-diabetic-effects-found-citrus-foods-and-juices.

Fitzpatrick, Kelly. "Superfood: Lemon." *Greatist*. March 6, 2012. http://greatist.com/health/superfood-lemon.

Hari, Vani. "Are You Making These Common Juicing Mistakes?" *Food Babe*. http://foodbabe.com/2013/08/05/juicing-mistakes.

Kadlovski, Shannon. "Five Foods That Kick Your Metabolism into Overdrive, Naturally!" *Huffington Post*. Updated March 6, 2012. http://www.huffingtonpost.ca/shannon-kadlovski/boost-metabolism-food_b_873851.html.

Lawless, Annie. "The pH Balance." *Blawnde*. http://www.blawnde.com/ph-balance.

Lawless, Annie. "Why Fats Are Phat." *Blawnde*. January 2, 2014. http://www.blawnde.com/fats-phat.

Lunger, Caroline. "Jump-Out the Toxins." *Gutsy*. January 14, 2013. http://www.mygutsy.com/jump-out-the-toxins-rebounding-for-lymph-drainage.

"Mint and Ginger Tea for Digestion." GrannyMed.com. http://www.grannymed.com/remedies/conditions/digestion/mint-and-ginger-tea-for-digestion.

Renz, Stacy. "Yoga and Digestion/Elimination." http://livingroomyoga.biz/yogastpetersburg/wp-content/uploads/2011/01/YOGA-AND-DIGESTION-and-ELIMINATION1.pdf.

Richards, Byron J. "Why Toxins and Waste Products Impede Weight Loss." Wellness Resources. April 16, 2012. http://www.wellnessresources.com/weight/articles/why_toxins_and_waste_products_impede_weight_loss_-_the_leptin_diet_weight_l.

Weil, Dr. Andrew. "Lymphatic Massage Therapy." DrWeil.com. http://www.drweil.com/drw/u/ART03409/Lymphatic-Massage-Therapy.html.

Young, Simon N. "How to Increase Serotonin in the Human Brain Without Drugs." *Journal of Psychiatry and Neuroscience* 32, no. 6 (November 2007): 394–99. http://www.ncbi.nlm.nih.gov/pmc/articles/PMC2077351.

CHAPTER 8. WEEK 2: 7 DAYS TO REINFORCE

"Beat Weight Loss with Healthy Beets." *Diet Bites*. http://www.dietbites.com/Diet-Articles-8/diet-beets.html.

Bianchi, Jane. "9 Habits That Slow Down Your Metabolism." *Redbook*. http://www.redbookmag.com/health-wellness/advice/slow-metabolism?click=main_sr#slide-1.

Dawson, Gloria, and Brian Clark Howard. "Top 10 Real Food Sources of Vitamin A." *Good Housekeeping*. http://www.goodhousekeeping.com/health/nutrition/vitamin-a-44010609.

Elias, Nina. "The #1 Food to Feel Full." *Prevention*. http://www.prevention.com/food/healthy-eating-tips/olive-oil-promotes-fullness.

Elkaim, Yuri, and Amy Coats. "Can You Exercise on a Cleanse?" Total Wellness Cleanse. http://totalwellnesscleanse.jimdo.com/can-you-exercise-while-on-a-cleanse.

Esser, William L. "Fruit Best Food of All." Raw Food Explained. http://www.rawfoodexplained.com/the-human-dietetic-character-part-ii/fruit-best-food-of-all.html.

Gueren, Casey. "7 Reasons to Work Out in the Morning." *Women's Health Magazine*. December 13, 2013. http://www.womenshealthmag.com/fitness/morning-exercise.

"How Does Your Liver Function to Cleanse and Detox Naturally?" Health Freedom Resources. http://healthfree.com/guide-to-liver-cleansing -detox-1.html.

Kelly, Diana. "The Best New Food for Diabetics." *Prevention*. http://www.prevention.com/food/ food-remedies/type-2-diabetics-can-improve -their-blood-sugar-beans.

Lawless, Annie. "The Guide to Healthy Oils." Suja Juice. April 21, 2014. http://www.sujajuice.com/ blog/the-guide-to-healthy-oils.

Lawless, Annie. "You Think It's Healthy but It's Lying, Part 1." *Blawnde*. September 8, 2014. http:// www.blawnde.com/healthy-lying-part.

Sheehan, Jan. "What Vitamins and Minerals Do Walnuts Have?" *SF Gate*. http://healthyeating .sfgate.com/vitamins-minerals-walnuts-have -4569.html.

Sisson, Mark. "Nuts and Omega-6s." *Mark's Daily Apple*. March 15, 2014. http://www.marksdailyapple.com/ nuts-omega-6-fats/#axzz3CbhdPvuu.

Wood, Rebecca. "Beans Build Energy." Rebecca Wood. http://www.rwood.com/Articles/Beans_ Build_Energy.htm.

Woodruff, Kary. "Eat Healthy Snacks During the Day to Prevent Overeating at Meals." Intermountain Healthcare. May 30, 2014. http:// intermountainhealthcare.org/blogs/2014/05/eat- healthy-snacks-during-the-day-to-prevent -overeating-at-meals.

CHAPTER 9. WEEK 3: 7 DAYS TO RECHARGE

Axe, Dr. Josh. "The Many Health Benefits of Raw Honey." Dr Axe. http://draxe.com/ the-many-health-benefits-of-raw-honey.

Beppu, F., M. Hosokawa, L. Tanaka, H. Kohno, T. Tanaka, and K. Miyashita. "Potent Inhibitory Effect of Trans9, Trans11 Isomer of Conjugated Linoleic Acid on the Growth of Human Colon Cancer Cells." *Journal of Nutritional Biochemistry* 17, no. 12 (December 2006): 830–36.

Bhattacharya, A., J. Banu, M. Rahman, J. Causey, and G. Fernandes. "Biological Effects of Conjugated Linoleic Acids in Health and Disease." *Journal of Nutritional Biochemistry* 17 (2006): 789–810.

Busch, Sandi. "The Health Benefits of Edamame." *SF Gate*. http://healthyeating.sfgate.com/health -benefits-edamame-1665.html.

Chengappa, M. M., and T. G. Nagaraja. "Liver Abscesses in Feedlot Cattle—A Review." *Journal of Animal Science* 76 (1998): 287–98.

Cooke, Dr. Thomas. "Benefits of Goat's Milk vs. Cow's Milk." Mt. Capra Wholefood Nutritionals. August 20, 2010. http://www.mtcapra.com/ benefits-of-goat-milk-vs-cow-milk.

Ehrlich, Steven D. "Manganese." University of Maryland Medical Center. http://umm.edu/health/ medical/altmed/supplement/manganese.

Federation of Quebec Maple Syrup Producers. "Benefits of Maple Syrup." Pure Canadian Maple Syrup. http://www.purecanadamaple.com/benefits-of-maple-syrup.

Felicetti, Marcus Julian. "11 Miraculous Ways Magnesium Heals Your Body and Mind." MindBodyGreen. July 16, 2012. http://www.mindbodygreen.com/0-5473/11-Miraculous-Ways-Magnesium-Heals-Your-Mind-Body.html.

Glick, Lila. "It's Official: Sugar Is the New Crack." TotalBeauty.com. http://www.totalbeauty.com/content/slideshows/natural-sugar-alternatives.

Goldberg, Max. "Move Over Coconut Water—Organic Green Juice Is the Best Post-Workout Drink." *Living Maxwell*. July 6, 2012. http://livingmaxwell.com/best-post-workout-drink.

"Got Milk?" Sheep 101. Updated May 27, 2012. http://www.sheep101.info/dairy.html.

Kelley, N. S., N. E. Hubbard, and K. L. Erickson. "Conjugated Linoleic Acid Isomers and Cancer." *Journal of Nutrition* 137, no. 12 (December 2007): 2599–607.

Kelly, Andrew P., and Eugene D. Janzen. "A Review of Morbidity and Mortality Rates and Disease Occurrence in North American Feedlot Cattle." *Canadian Veterinary Journal* 27, no. 12 (December 1986): 496–500.

Kresser, Chris. "Why Grass-Fed Trumps Grain-Fed." Chris Kresser. http://chriskresser.com/why-grass-fed-trumps-grain-fed.

Lipman, Dr. Frank. "Feel Good Fast: Let Go of Gluten." Dr. Frank Lipman. http://www.drfranklipman.com/feel-good-fast-let-go-of-gluten.

Phillips, K. M., M. H. Carlsen, and R. Blomhoff. "Total Antioxidant Content of Alternatives to Refined Sugar." *Journal of the American Dietetic Association* 109, no. 1 (January 2009): 64–71. doi:10.1016/j.jada.2008.10.014.

Siemens, Michael. "Tools for Optimizing Feedlot Production." University of Wisconsin–Extension. 1996. http://learningstore.uwex.edu/assets/pdfs/A3661.pdf.

Sterling, Kathryn. "Processed Gluten Free Foods Can Be Hazardous to Your Health, Not Helpful, Experts Say." *Pittsburgh Post-Gazette*. November 4, 2013. http://www.post-gazette.com/frontpage/2013/11/04/DIET-S-DOWNSIDE/stories/201311040018.

CHAPTER 10. WEEK 4: 7 DAYS TO RENEW

Appleton, Nancy. *Lick the Sugar Habit*, 2nd ed. New York: Avery, 1988.

Gaudreau, Stephanie. "Why Peanuts Make People Go Crazy." *Stupid Easy Paleo*. October 24, 2013. http://stupideasypaleo.com/2013/10/24/why-peanuts-make-people-go-crazy.

Lawless, Annie. "How to Break Up with Processed Foods." *Blawnde*. March 24, 2014. http://www.blawnde.com/break-processed-foods.

Lawless, Annie. "You Think It's Healthy but It's Lying, Part V." *Blawnde*. June 20, 2014. http://www.blawnde.com/healthy-lying-part-2.

Mercola, Dr. "Soy: This Miracle Health Food Has Been Linked to Brain Damage and Breast Cancer." Mercola. September 18, 2010. http://articles.mercola.com/sites/articles/archive/2010/09/18/soy-can-damage-your-health.aspx.

Michaelis, Kristen. "Agave Nectar: Good or Bad?" *Food Renegade*. January 7, 2010. http://www.foodrenegade.com/agave-nectar-good-or-bad.

Turay, Mariam. "Why Juice? Juicing Benefits." April 13, 2012. http://www.greenjuiceaday.com/juicing-benefits.

Williams, Dr. David. "Beneficial Bacteria for Digestive and Overall Health." Dr. David Williams. Updated April 17, 2014. http://www.drdavidwilliams.com/beneficial-bacteria-aid-health.

Zelman, Kathleen M. "The Truth About White Foods." *WebMD*. http://www.webmd.com/diet/features/truth-about-white-foods.

CHAPTER 11. THE SUJA LIFESTYLE

Dalen, J., B. W. Smith, B. M. Shelley, A. L. Sloan, L. Leahigh, and D. Begay. "Pilot Study: Mindful Eating and Living (MEAL): Weight, Eating Behavior, and Psychological Outcomes Associated with a Mindfulness-Based Intervention for People with Obesity." *Complementary Therapies in Medicine* 18, no. 6 (2010): 260–64.

Dulan, Mitzi. "6 Benefits to Being a Morning Exerciser." *U.S. News and World Report*. Updated September 27, 2013. http://www.huffingtonpost.com/2013/09/27/when-to-exercise_n_3982906.html.

Fung, Maple M., Katherine Peters, Susan Redline, Michael G. Ziegler, Sonia Ancoli-Israel, Elizabeth Barrett-Connor, and Katie L. Stone. "Decreased Slow Wave Sleep Increases Risk of Developing Hypertension in Elderly Men." *Hypertension*. April 10, 2011. http://hyper.ahajournals.org/content/early/2011/08/28/HYPERTENSIONAHA.111.174409.abstrac.

Glozier, Nicholas, Alexandra Martiniuk, George Patton, Rebecca Ivers, Qiang Li, Ian Hickie, MD, Teresa Senserrick, Mark Woodward, Robyn Norton, and Mark Stevenson. "Short Sleep Duration and Psychological Distress in Young Adults." *Sleep*. http://www.journalsleep.org/ViewAbstract.aspx?pid=27892.

Haiken, Melanie. "Jet Lag, Late Nights, and Naps Disrupt Gene Function, New Study Shows." *Forbes*. January 22, 2014. http://www.forbes.com/sites/melaniehaiken/2014/01/22/jet-lag-and-working-at-night-disrupts-your-genes-new-study-shows.

Harvard School of Public Health. "Waking Up to Sleep's Role in Weight Control." *Obesity Prevention Source*. http://www.hsph.harvard.edu/obesity-prevention-source/obesity-causes/sleep-and-obesity.

Jequier, E. "Alcohol Intake and Body Weight: A Paradox." *American Journal of Clinical Nutrition* 69 (1999): 173–74.

King, Peter. "Study: Light Exercise Has Big Health Benefits." *Newsday*. May 23, 2014. http://www.newsday.com/lifestyle/retirement/study-light-exercise-has-big-health-benefits-1.8162296.

Kristeller, Jean L., and C. Brendan Hallett. "An Exploratory Study of a Meditation-Based Intervention for Binge Eating Disorder." *Journal of Health Psychology* 4, no. 3 (1999): 357–63.

Mattes, Richard D. "Hunger and Thirst: Issues in Measurement and Prediction of Eating and Drinking." *Physiology and Behavior* 100, no. 1 (April 26, 2010): 22–32.

Suter, P. M., E. Hasler, and W. Vetter. "Effects of Alcohol on Energy Metabolism and Body Weight Regulation: Is Alcohol a Risk Factor for Obesity?" *Nutrition Review* 55 (1997): 157–71.

Suter, P. M., Y. Schutz, and E. Jéquier. "The Effect of Ethanol on Fat Storage in Healthy Subjects." *New England Journal of Medicine* 326 (1992): 983–87.

Wannamethee, S., and A. G. Shaper. "Alcohol, Body Weight and Weight Gain in Middle-Aged Men." *American Journal of Clinical Nutrition* 77, no. 5 (2003): 1312–17.

Wright, Brierley. "6 Benefits of Staying Hydrated." August 8, 2012. *One:Life*. http://www.onemedical.com/blog/live-well/6-benefits-of-staying-hydrated.

PART 3. RECIPES

Adams, Mike. "Miso." Healing Food Reference. http://www.healingfoodreference.com/miso.html.

Campbell, Meg. "Soluble Fiber in Sweet Potatoes." *SF Gate*. http://healthyeating.sfgate.com/soluble-fiber-sweet-potatoes-6416.html.

"Chickpeas." Natural Food Benefits. http://www.naturalfoodbenefits.com/display.asp?CAT=2&ID=86.

"Coconut Secrets for Optimal Health." Coconut Secret. https://www.coconutsecret.com/coconuthealthsecrets2.html.

"Coconut." Coconut Research Center. http://www.coconutresearchcenter.org.

Daniluk, Julie. "Crush Your Cravings with 5 Appetite Suppressing Foods." *The Doctor Oz Show*. May 25, 2011. http://www.doctoroz .com/article/crush-your-cravings-5-appetite -suppressing-foods.

Dumas, Kiley. "6 Health Benefits of Eating Beets." Full Circle. http://www.fullcircle.com/ goodfoodlife/2012/05/10/6-health-benefits-of -eating-beets.

"Easy Metabolism Boosting Tips." CBS News. September 2, 2008. http://www.cbsnews.com/ news/easy-metabolism-boosting-tips.

Enig, Mary. "A New Look at Coconut Oil." The Weston A. Price Foundation. http:// www.westonaprice.org/health-topics/ a-new-look-at-coconut-oil.

Fitzpatrick, Kelly. "Superfood: Lemon." *Greatist*. http://greatist.com/health/superfood-lemon.

Fredenburg, May. "Cucumber and Electrolytes." *SF Gate*. http://healthyeating.sfgate.com/cucumber -electrolytes-10852.html.

Group, Dr. Edward F. "17 Health Benefits of Cayenne Pepper." Global Healing Center. Updated May 5, 2014. http://www.globalhealingcenter.com/ natural-health/benefits-of-cayenne-pepper.

Gunnars, Kris. "6 Proven Benefits of Apple Cider Vinegar." *Authority Nutrition*. http:// authoritynutrition.com/6-proven-health-benefits -of-apple-cider-vinegar.

Gunnars, Kris. "10 Proven Health Benefits of Turmeric and Curcumin." *Authority Nutrition*. http://authoritynutrition.com/top-10-evidence -based-health-benefits-of-turmeric.

Gunnars, Kris. "11 Proven Health Benefits of Chia Seeds." *Authority Nutrition*. http:// authoritynutrition.com/11-proven-health -benefits-of-chia-seeds.

Gutierre, David. "The Secret Healing Benefits of Miso." *Natural News*. July 30, 2012. http://www .naturalnews.com/036618_miso_fermented_ food_nutrition.html.

"The Healing Power of Betalains." *Wellness Guy*. May 18, 2011. http://wellnessguide4u.blogspot .com/2011/05/healing-power-of-betalains.html.

"Health Benefits of Cabbage." Organic Facts. https://www.organicfacts.net/health-benefits/ vegetable/health-benefits-of-cabbage.html.

"Health Benefits of Lime." Organic Facts. https:// www.organicfacts.net/health-benefits/fruit/ health-benefits-of-lime.ht.

"Health Benefits of Oats." Whole Grains Council. http://wholegrainscouncil.org/whole-grains-101/ health-benefits-of-oats.

"How to Raise Metabolism." eMedExpert. Last updated March 1, 2014. http://www.emedexpert .com/tips/metabolism-tips.shtml.

Kanner, J., S. Haril, and R. Granit. "Betalains: A New Class of Dietary Cationized Antioxidants." *Journal of Agricultural and Food Chemistry* 49, no. 11 (November 2001): 5178–85. http://www.ncbi.nlm.nih.gov/pubmed/11714300.

Kim, Dr. Ben. "Calcium Rich Plant Foods Better for Bones than Dairy." Dr. Ben Kim. http://drbenkim.com/recipestahinidressing.html.

Lawless, Annie. "Carrots—Not Just for Rabbits." Suja Juice. June 26, 2013. http://www.sujajuice.com/blog/carrots-not-just-for-rabbits.

Lawless, Annie. "Foods That Are Actually Healthy." *Blawnde*. September 8, 2014. http://www.blawnde.com/foods-that-are-actually-healthy.

Layton, Julia. "How Does Dietary Fat Help Us Absorb Vitamins?" How Stuff Works. http://health.howstuffworks.com/wellness/food-nutrition/vitamin-supplements/fat-absorb-vitamins.htm.

"Lentils: A Savory Way to Steady Blood Sugar." Share Care. January 2010. http://www.sharecare.com/health/type-2-diabetes/article/blood-sugar-benefits-lentils.

Lewin, Jo. "The Health Benefits of...Salmon." *BBC GoodFood*. http://www.bbcgoodfood.com/howto/guide/ingredient-focus-salmon.

Magee, Elaine. "The Benefits of Flaxseed." *WebMD*. http://www.webmd.com/diet/features/benefits-of-flaxseed.

Marie, Joanne. "Antioxidant Benefits of Raw Cacao." *SF Gate*. http://healthyeating.sfgate.com/antioxidant-benefits-raw-cacao-3990.html.

Matheny, Monica. "The Ultimate Guide to Oats." The Yummy Life. http://www.theyummylife.com/Oats.

Mercola, Dr. "What Are the Health Benefits of Carrots?" Mercola. December 28, 2013. http://articles.mercola.com/sites/articles/archive/2013/12/28/carrot-health-benefits.aspx.

Mitchell, Lisa. "15 Reasons to Use Apple Cider Vinegar Every Day." MindBodyGreen. http://www.mindbodygreen.com/0-5875/15-Reasons-to-Use-Apple-Cider-Vinegar-Every-Day.html.

Swenson, Sam. "5 Ways to Add Lemon to Your Diet." Suja Juice. June 6, 2014. http://www.sujajuice.com/blog/5-ways-to-add-lemon-to-your-diet.

Swenson, Sam. "6 Super Sources of Omega-3s." Suja Juice. August 12, 2014. http://www.sujajuice.com/blog/6-super-sources-of-omega-3-s.

Swenson, Sam. "8 Foods Women Should Eat Everyday." Suja Juice. August 7, 2014. http://www.sujajuice.com/blog/8-foods-women-should-eat-everyday.

Swenson, Sam. "Complete Meat-Free Proteins." Suja Juice. January 28, 2014. http://www.sujajuice.com/blog/complete-meat-free-proteins.

"Top 10 Foods Highest in Vitamin A." HealthAliciousNess. http://www.healthaliciousness.com/articles/food-sources-of-vitamin-A.php.

Tremblay, Louise. "Nutrients and Benefits of Chick Peas and Garbanzo Beans." *SF Gate*. http://healthyeating.sfgate.com/nutrients-benefits-chick-peas-garbanzo-beans-7490.html.

Tsakos, Lisa. "8 Reasons to Start Your Day with Lemon Water." *Naturally Savvy*. October 10, 2013. http://naturallysavvy.com/eat/8-reasons-to-start-your-day-with-lemon-water.

Tyler, Mara. "10 Vegan Sources of Protein." MindBodyGreen. May 10, 2012. http://www.mindbodygreen.com/0-4771/10-Vegan-Sources-of-Protein.html.

Upton, Julie. "Benefits of Beets." Suja Juice. June 26, 2014. http://www.sujajuice.com/blog/benefits-of-beets.

Upton, Julie. "Crazy for Coconuts." Suja Juice. April 15, 2014. http://www.sujajuice.com/blog/crazy-for-coconuts.

Upton, Julie. "The Power of Turmeric." Suja Juice. April 10, 2014. http://www.sujajuice.com/blog/the-power-of-turmeric.

Upton, Julie. "Turn Up the Heat with Cayenne Pepper." Suja Juice. March 18, 2014. http://www.sujajuice.com/blog/turn-up-the-heat-with-cayenne-pepper.

Ware, Megan. "What Are the Health Benefits of Mint?" *MNT*. Updated August 30, 2014. http://www.medicalnewstoday.com/articles/275944.php.

Weil, Dr. Andrew. "3 Reasons to Eat Turmeric." DrWeil.com. http://www.drweil.com/drw/u/ART03001/Three-Reasons-to-Eat-Turmeric.html.

"Why You Should Eat More Wheat Berries." *The Kitchn*. http://www.thekitchn.com/chewy-nutty-nutritious-wheat-berries-ingredient-spotlight-176749.

Young, Lesley. "5 Superfoods That Help You Slim Down." *Canadian Living*. http://www.freshjuice.ca/eat-well/everyday-healthy-eating/5-superfoods-that-help-you-slim-down/s/779/3.

INDEX

· ·